BDSM Basics for Beginners

A Guide for Dominants and Submissives Starting to Explore the Lifestyle

Michelle Fegatofi

3/13/2013

BDSM Basics for Beginners – A guide for Dominants and Submissives Starting to Explore the Lifestyle
Second Edition

Copyright © 2013 Michelle Fegatofi
ISBN 978-1-300-83710-7

1

First and foremost, this book is dedicated to Padrone. Without all of your help, guidance, wisdom, encouragement and most of all - love, I know I would never have been able to accomplish all that I have so far. Thank you amore mio. Ti amo.

To all my loyal readers and internet fans, thanks for all the questions and inspirational messages from you all. You are the ones that made me want to write a comprehensive, but easy to understand, beginners guide in the first place.

- Michelle

Contents

Introduction

Now that you have taken the first step into the wide world of BDSM, let me be the first to welcome you to this wonderful, very fulfilling journey.

Take the time to explore all the variations of roles, relationships and scene play within the Lifestyle. Explore whether you are a Top (Dominant) or a bottom (submissive), or if you enjoy playing both roles, known as a Switch. Whichever role you pick, research that role and gain a working knowledge before you actually participate in any play sessions. This way, you have a better understanding of how different roles work and a basic understanding of rules and protocols that exist for that role.

There are many levels to Dominance and submission. The first thing I want you to know is that there is no "right way" to participate in or practice BDSM. Always keep an open mind and remember to never judge others. Just because something might be a kink you are not into, does not mean that it is wrong.

Make the experience what you and your partner wants. Follow the rule SSC (Safe, Sane, Consensual) or RACK (Risk Aware Consensual Kink). Make sure you have a solid idea of what you want out of BDSM and do your homework before participating in any activities. Always remember, knowledge is power.

In the following pages, I will try to lay out the basics of BDSM from the text book standpoint, but will also give you more insights into my own daily life and routine, rules I have to follow, and the form of submission that we prefer to practice. As I stated earlier, the way you choose to practice or live BDSM comes from what you and your partner choose. There is no right or wrong as long as both of you agree and follow the rules and guidelines set up before entering into a relationship.

I hope reading the 'text book' versions and definitions, as well as the glimpses of my own life I provide throughout the book, gives each of you a broader understanding and helps to guide you further on your own journey into practicing your own version of the Lifestyle.

Chapter One

What is BDSM?

What is BDSM and what does BDSM stand for? There are many variations of what the initials BDSM stand for, but the most widely used is Bondage, Discipline, Sadism, and Masochism. When grouped together, BDSM springs from the terms Bondage and Discipline (B/D), Dominance and Submission (D/s), and Sadism and Masochism (S/M) and describes forms of sexuality that incorporate restraint, pressure, sensation, training, and elements of both erotic and non-erotic power exchange.

Generally, it is used as an umbrella term for a consenting adult relationship that involves a power exchange. For example, in a Dominant/submissive relationship, the Dominant person holds authority over the submissive person. Because of the inequality of these roles, it is important that both adults have discussed, negotiated, and consented to their defined roles.

Bondage is any kind of item used to restrain any part of a sub/slave's body. Most commonly used restraints are toy handcuffs, rope, or some type of quick release or Velcro closing restraint.

Discipline is the actions taken by a Dominant to teach and prevent a submissive from doing something that is in no way an act of willful disobedience. Discipline does not normally include physical punishment.

Punishment is when a submissive or slave has purposely been disobedient and has knowingly disobeyed a command or done something incorrectly brought on by an act of defiance. In cases like these, punishment will be administered to ensure that the submissive or slave is aware that disobedience has consequences and it generally is not a process that any of the parties involved, enjoys. I will touch on this more in depth later in this book.

Sadism is a source of pleasure that results from inflicting pain or humiliation or watching pain or humiliation inflicted on a submissive/slave.

Masochism is a source of sexual/mental/emotional gratification, or the tendency to derive sexual/mental/emotional gratification, from being physically or emotionally abused.

BDSM is a sexual preference and a form of personal relationship. It is also extremely mental, but even more so to those that practice it in situations other than sexual scenes. Interest in BDSM can range from one-time experimentation to a Lifestyle. A Dominant has to be very careful and know his submissive extremely well in order not to do any lasting mental damage if the sub is deep into submission.

Many people practice some element of BDSM in their sexual lives without even necessarily being aware of it. They may think of S&M as "That sick stuff that people do with whips and cattle prods and stuff," yet still blindfold one another from time to time, or tie one another down and break out the whipped cream. All of these things are BDSM.

BDSM is not necessarily hardcore sadomasochism. It can be remarkably subtle and sensual and soft. Pinning your partner to the bed and running silk or ice cubes or rabbit fur over your lover's body also qualifies as BDSM, specifically, of a variety called sensation play.

BDSM is **NOT** abuse. An abuser doesn't take the time to learn safe play and an abuser certainly doesn't respect limits. Not taking NO for an answer, not honoring a safe word, or taking advantage of the unequal power relationship that exists between Dom and sub, are forms of abuse. While these relationships do not fit into the traditional mold, they are between consenting adults. If one person withdraws their consent, it could become abuse, but that can also happen in a vanilla relationship as well.

To gauge how a scene is going, those in the Community may use safewords to check in with each other. "Green" means that everything is going well, so whatever activity is going on can continue or get more intense. "Yellow" means to slow down or take a break. "Red" means stop immediately.

This is where knowledge comes in handy and trust is essential. Never play or submit to anyone that you do not completely trust with that power.

Is BDSM Normal?

Normal is defined as conforming to the standard or the common type; usual; not abnormal; regular. Normality is an idealistic state of living, of existing. Since normality varies from person to person, culture to culture, and decade to decade, any recognized standard will always be whatever practices and lifestyles the current Mainstream society decides amongst the confirmed members of each class, to be 'Normal'. You have to think, one person's morality is different from another, so that would make what you consider normal different from me or even your neighbor's version of normal.

If we view BDSM from the view point of the current world's population, then no it is not considered normal. Think about the sexual practices in the BDSM Lifestyle (Bondage, S&M, Poly, Swinging, etc...). Main stream culture usually follows some type of religious teachings (Jewish, Catholic, Muslim, Buddist, etc...) that teach sex is only supposed to be used for procreation. They frown on anything outside their strict religious codes. They consider bondage or flogging abuse. But, people that practice these and other forms of sexual torture within the confines of the BDSM lifestyle, get heightened pleasure and love the bite of the whip on their back or the pinch of clamps on their nipples. Is it normal? For some yes, for others, no. Again, it depends on your perception of Normality.

Main stream western culture would also consider any type submission (in males or females) weird, or not normal, because most of the population now consider males and females equal in most settings. They ask why would one person want to give over any freedoms, allow anyone else to make any decisions for them, or submit to another person's will. They don't understand the sense of security, need of serving, and feelings of yearning to be dominated and/or owned by another individual. I don't mean in a creepy, stalker, or 1800's kind of way. For most submissives or slaves in the Lifestyle, they will tell you that they find more freedom and happiness in being owned, being given rules and regulations, having to follow certain standards and guidelines, than they do in typical or 'vanilla' relationships.

I consider a BDSM Lifestyle normal, because I chose to practice this type of Lifestyle as a 24/7 consensual slave. Whether my Padrone (Master) is with me or not, I always follow his guidelines and rules. I gain extreme satisfaction and peace of mind and spirit by the rules and guidelines he has set for me. I have a very deep sense of love and protection all the time and that gives me a happiness that is almost indescribable.

So, is BDSM normal? Yes and No. Since normality is relative, you have to decide.

BDSM vs Abuse – What to Watch Out For

If you feel threatened in a bad way, if your submission is forced or something about the relationship makes you think or feel bad all the time and you get no comfort from it, it is more likely abuse than a BDSM relationship.

Telling the Difference between Consensual BDSM and abuse:

1. Restraints. Abusers tend to restrain their victims with fear and intimidation, not safety clips and quick releases.
2. The availability of mentors, reference materials and technical guides.
3. SM rarely results in facial marks or marks that are received on the forearms (defensive marks).
4. There is usually an even pattern of marks if it is SM, indicating the bottom held quite still during the stimulation.
5. The marks are often quite well-defined when inflicted by a toy like cane or whip, whereas in abuse there are blotches of soft-tissue bruising, randomly distributed.
6. The common areas for SM stimulation is on the buttocks, thighs, back, breasts, or the genitals. The fleshy parts of the body can be stimulated intensely and pleasurably.
7. D/s is about the building of a trusting relationship between two consenting adult partners.
8. Abuse is about the breach of trust between an authority figure and the person in their care.
9. D/s is about the mutual respect demonstrated between two enlightened people.
10. Abuse is about the lack of respect that one person demonstrates to another person.
11. D/s is about a shared enjoyment of controlled erotic pain and/or humiliation for mutual pleasure.
12. Abuse is about a form of out-of-control physical violence and/or personal or emotional degradation of the submissive.
13. D/s is about loving each other completely and without reservation in an alternate way.
14. Abuse is hurtful. It is also very damaging emotionally and spiritually to the submissive.
15. D/s frees a submissive from the restraints of years of vanilla conditioning to explore a buried part of herself.

16. Abuse binds a submissive to a lonely and solitary life of shame, fear and secrecy... imprisoning her very soul.
17. D/s builds self-esteem as a person discovers and embraces their long hidden sexuality.
18. Abuse shatters and destroys a person's self-esteem and leaves self-hatred in its place.

Chapter Two

Historical Origins of BDSM

The historical origins of BDSM are obscure. During the ninth century BC, ritual flagellations were performed in Artemis Orthia, one of the most important religious areas of ancient Sparta, where the Cult of Orthia, a preolympic religion, was practiced. Here, ritual flagellation called diamastigosis took place on a regular basis.

One of the oldest graphical proofs of sadomasochistic activities is found in an Etruscan burial site in Tarquinia. Inside the Tomba della Fustigazione (Flogging grave), in the latter sixth century b.c., two men are portrayed flagellating a woman with a cane and a hand during an erotic situation. Another reference related to flagellation is to be found in the sixth book of the Satires of the ancient Roman Poet Juvenal (1st–2nd century A.D.). Further reference can be found in Petronius's Satyricon where a delinquent is whipped for sexual arousal. Anecdotal narratives related to humans who have had themselves voluntary bound, flagellated or whipped as a substitute for sex or as part of foreplay reach back to the third and fourth century.

The Kama Sutra describes four different kinds of hitting during lovemaking, the allowed regions of the human body to target and different kinds of joyful "cries of pain" practiced by bottoms. The collection of historic texts related to sensuous experiences explicitly emphasizes that impact play, biting and pinching during sexual activities should only be performed consensually since only some women consider such behavior to be joyful. From this perspective, the Kama Sutra can be considered as one of the first written resources dealing with sadomasochistic activities and safety rules.

Further texts with sadomasochistic connotation appear worldwide during the following centuries on a regular basis. There are reports of people willingly being bound or whipped, as a prelude to or substitute for sex, during the fourteenth century. The medieval phenomenon of courtly love in all of its slavish devotion and ambivalence has been suggested by some writers to be a precursor of BDSM. Some sources claim that BDSM as a distinct form of sexual behavior originated at the beginning of the eighteenth century when Western civilization began medically and legally categorizing sexual behavior. There are reports of brothels specializing in flagellation as early as 1769, and John Cleland's novel Fanny Hill, published in 1749, mentions a flagellation scene. Other sources give a broader definition, citing BDSM-like behavior in earlier times and other cultures, such as the medieval flagellates and the physical ordeal rituals of some Native American societies.

Although the names of the Marquis de Sade and Leopold von Sacher-Masoch are attached to the terms sadism and masochism respectively, Sade's way of life does not meet modern BDSM standards of informed consent. BDSM ideas and imagery have existed on the fringes of Western culture throughout the twentieth century. Robert Bienvenu attributes the origins of modern BDSM to three sources, which he names as "European Fetish" (from 1928), "American Fetish" (from 1934), and "Gay Leather" (from 1950). Another source are the sexual games played in brothels, which go back into the nineteenth century if not earlier. Irving Klaw, during the 1950s and 1960s, produced some of the first commercial film and photography with a BDSM theme (most notably with Bettie Page) and published comics by the now-iconic bondage artists John Willie and Eric Stanton.

Stanton's model Bettie Page became one of the first successful models in the area of fetish photography and one of the most famous pin-up girls of American mainstream culture. Italian author and designer Guido Crepax was deeply influenced by him, coining the style and development of European adult comics in the second half of the twentieth century. The artists Helmut Newton and Robert Mapplethorpe are the most prominent examples of the increasing use of BDSM-related motives in modern photography and the public discussions still resulting from this.

Now that you understand more of the historical origins, you probably also know that there has been yet another addition to the evolution of BDSM, via the internet. There are two ways now that you can practice a BDSM Lifestyle - Real Life (commonly RL for short) and Cyber (internet and/or some other kind of technological connection). Most people that live the Lifestyle in RL do not think that Cyber BDSM is a real form of BDSM because there is no physical contact. But I disagree. If the connection and trust is there between two people, it can be very real to both of them, even without the physical contact. BDSM in this case is 100% mental. It is about the satisfaction both parties receive from their chosen role (Dominating or submitting). I have devoted an entire chapter to that of Cyber BDSM.

Chapter Three

Commonly Used Terms

Now you have a better understanding of what BDSM is and what it is not, let's cover some basic terms that you are most likely to hear when speaking or reading about the Lifestyle. I have already used some previously.

Top/Dominant/Dom/Domme
These titles refer to the person in charge or in control; the one that must be obeyed. Domme (usually pronounced "doe-may") is a female Dominant.
These titles are generally used when referring to relationships that are not defined as Full Time roles, but used only during scenes or within a BDSM setting.

Master/Mistress
These titles refer to the dominant person or the one in control in a Master/slave relationship, usually defined as a Full Time D/s relationship. This can refer to a couple that live together and practice the roles 24/7, or it can also be two people that always enter into their specified role when they are together.

Bottom/Submissive
These titles refer to a person who gives up control and gets emotional or sexual satisfaction from aspects of submission which may include serving or being used by the Dominant.

Slave
This title refers to the deepest level of submission. A slave is an individual who is wholly under the control and or power of a Master or Dominant. They freely surrendered their rights and privileges as an individual, and forfeited the ability to act as an independent entity. A slave is the property of their Master, this includes all of their belongings as well as their bodies and emotions. A slave thrives on the opportunity to provide unconditional service and to exceed their Owner's expectations. The slave is devoted to the service and the will of their Owner and feels the need deep within them. They are usually most happy when their Owner is happy.

Switch
This title refers to someone who plays both Dom and Sub roles, usually with different partners.

Consent
Mutual agreement to the terms of a scene or ongoing BDSM relationship.

DM
Dungeon Monitor/Master - a person who volunteers to supervise the interactions between participants at a play party to ensure their safety.

D/s
Domination/submission

Dungeon
Usually referring to a room or area with BDSM equipment. Can be a synonym for play room.

Fetish
A specific obsession or delight in one object or experience.

Munch
A group of people that are into BDSM meeting at a vanilla place.

Newbie
Someone new to BDSM.

Negotiation
The consensual agreements between Top and Bottom, spoken or written in contract form, outlining Hard Limits, punishments, and expected behavior.

Play Party
A BDSM event involving many people engaging in Scenes.

Protocol(s)

Written or unwritten "rules" and guidelines that are followed by BDSM participants. Most commonly used in strict 24/7 relationships.

RACK

Risk-aware consensual kink. Used by some of the Community to describe a philosophical view that is generally permissive of certain risky sexual behaviors, as long as the participants are fully aware of the risks.

SSC

Safe, sane and consensual
SAFE: attempts should be made to identify and prevent risks to health
SANE: activities should be undertaken in a sane and sensible state of mind
CONSENTUAL: all activities should involve the fully informed consent of all parties involved.

Safeword

When a participant utters a safeword, ALL activity stops; either completely or to reframe and renegotiate the scene. "Red" is the most common.

Scene

"a scene" refers to the time period of BDSM activities.
"The Scene" refers to the entire lifestyle of being involved in BDSM.

Subspace

A mental altered state in which a person can be taken to. Space is a form of hypnotism that can be self-attained, or a Dominant can aid to obtain. Subspace is used for sexual pleasure, and can be utilized to convert pain to pleasure. After care is mandatory, as is constant monitoring. Not for the novice.

Vanilla

Someone or something which does not encompass BDSM activity.

Wannabe

Someone who thinks or claims to be knowledgeable about BDSM, but is not. Especially prevalent with new Doms.

Chapter Four

Limits and Safewords

If you have been around or explored the world of BDSM for any length of time, you will have heard of Limits. If you have no clue as to what the true meaning of Limits is, the easiest explanation I can give you is this: Limits encompass everything (mentally, physically, emotionally) that you will and will not allow in a BDSM relationship.

It is important to note that scene play does not have to involve all forms of BDSM. Some Dominant/submissive relationships are purely intellectual. There really is no right or wrong way to play, as long as safety isn't ignored.

Do your homework and read as much as you can about different aspects of BDSM scene play, bondage, and roles. The more informed you are, the better you can decide what you are more comfortable with.

If you are at a place that you are thinking of entering into a BDSM contract with someone, you have to have all of your limits in place and make sure they will be honored by your Dominant. Write down 3 lists, one that contains things that are permissible, one that contains things that you may want to try but are scared to, and one that contains items that are absolutely off limits, no matter what your Dominant says or does.

Before a BDSM scene, it is common for participants to negotiate an outline of what activities will and will not take place during the play session. At this stage, participants outline what they want to happen and hard and soft limits are determined. For example, it is common to set a time limit on the session, to set a safeword and to prohibit activity involving non-consenting 3rd parties.

Hard Limits
Something that must not be done. Violating a hard limit is often considered just cause for ending a scene or even a relationship.

Soft Limits
Something that someone will do only in special circumstances or when highly aroused.

Safeword
Safewords are intended to protect participants from going further or doing things they don't wish to do. Safewords are also intended to end or slow down the scene for other reasons, such as a cramp, charley horse or a sudden onset of dizziness or shortness of breath.

The whole point of choosing a safeword is to select a word that you would not normally use in conversation, not even in animated conversation. Choosing a word like *Stop* or *Ow* wouldn't work because often, stop doesn't mean stop, it means 'if you stop now I will scream!' and 'Ow' can mean 'this is so yummy, please may I have another?' Choosing *Elephant* or *Babysitter*, *Frog legs* or *Chicken* as your safeword is a much better idea. Ok, chicken fried steak might be too hard to remember, so maybe stick with the one word safewords. I mean, really, how often do you think a person is tied to a St. Andrew's Cross enjoying the flogger so much they are flying into subspace and the word babysitter comes to their mind?

The Myth of Safewords is that a safeword will protect the submissive from harm. That is utter crap! A safeword has absolutely no power to protect the submissive from harm. In fact, I believe that trusting in safewords can often create a false sense of safety for submissives. A submissive is falsely comforted by the Top's giving them a safeword. The safeword is of no value whatsoever, without knowing and trusting the Top, and how in the world could a submissive possibly trust someone they spent a total of a few hours on the internet with, prior to agreeing to play with them?

Safewords are usually agreed upon before playing a scene by all participants, and many organized BDSM groups have standard safewords that all members agree to use to avoid confusion at organized play events.

Chapter Five

Varieties of Toys and Implements Used in BDSM

Below is a list of different kinds of play. Please note that they all can utilize mental and/or physical play.

Age Play
Acting as if you younger or perhaps older than you really are.

Anal Beads
A set of strung beads used to insert into the anus to stimulate the anal nerves as foreplay or to cause orgasm.

Anal Play
This is generally play where the anus may be penetrated with either beads, ice, dildos, anal plugs, penis, or fist. Rimming the anus with a finger or toys stimulates the nerves which can create a more intense orgasm. Inserting and playing with one's prostate gland (males) will cause increased orgasm.

Animal Role Playing
Games in which one or more partners, usually the bottom, takes on the role of an animal. Most common is probably a dog, though horses are also popular. The 'animal' may imitate animal behavior, wear items such as collars, leads, bridles and so on, or carry out tasks associated with animal behavior.

Ball Stretching
Play which involves a type of penile constraint attached to weights in order to provide a variety of sensations including discomfort and pain, while stretching the testicles and scrotum.

Bathroom Use Control

Scenes where the Dominant restricts or takes control over the submissive's bodily functions through the use of techniques such as catheterization, enemas, diapers, rubber pants, and possibly golden showers. Examples in play: House training a puppy, age play, and golden shower play.

Beating

Striking the body with various objects or the hand. Typically administered as punishment in connection with childhood punishments. For example, the Dominant may administer a "beating" to an unruly submissive.

Being serviced (sexually)

The Dominant instructing the submissive to do exactly how He / She wants the submissive to perform sexually.

Blindfolds

Play which involves temporarily blocking the submissive's sense of sight. This type of play is essential when everyday objects are used to give unexpected sensations. Blindfolds come in many forms from the more expensive leather (full-head type) to the more inexpensive handkerchiefs, scarves, bandages. Safety Note: Do not make the blindfold too tight as to put pressure on the eyeballs. Although some people take blindfolding in stride, it can have unpredictable psychological effects and be extremely frightening for some people.

Boot Worship

The practice of play involving a fetish for boots / shoes. Commonly used for Domination and humiliation practices (i.e., licking or cleaning of the Dominant's boots, shoes or bare feet).

Bondage

The restriction of a person's bodily movements for erotic reasons using fastenings of various types or textures. Also used in S/m practices though with a heavier pretense. Examples; Rope, cuffs, chains, and other restraining devices.

Cages

Most common is the use of a large animal cage. Construction of a cage can be of wood, steel, fencing material. Used to confine the submissive, for play or punishment.

Caning

Mostly made of bamboo, this whip is by far the most painful. Care should be used, as the welts from caning are slow to rise, and blood can be accidentally drawn if not in constant monitoring. Caning should be limited to the fleshy part of the buttocks, and nowhere else on the body. This can be very dangerous, and is not for the novice.

Chastity Belt

In S/m circles, meaning the banning or physically preventing one (male or female) from achieving orgasm or any form of genital stimulation. A means of domination over one's submissive.
A device (lockable) panty-type which when worn prevents any type of genital stimulation.

Clothespins

Generally used in BDSM play as quite effective nipple clamps, testicle clamps, etc. Be sure the wood doesn't become stuck to the skin while removing, as it will remove skin from body.

Cock & Ball Torture

Any form of restraint or orgasm control to a male's genitals. Can be used for play or punishment. Not for the novice, as this can be dangerous.

Cock Worship

Play which involves the fantasy of worshiping the cock. Performed mostly by the submissive to the Dominant. Scenes might include licking and / or fellatio.

Collar

A collar worn around the neck to indicate one's submissiveness. These can be made of leather, steel, rubber, rope. Used in scenes for humiliation and / or examples such as dog / puppy or even boy / girl play.

Cuffs

A leather or metal bondage device used to restrict movement. Usually locks around the limbs in order to place the submissive in a precarious position.

Dildo
They may be hand-held, strapped on with harnesses to allow women to wear, or permanently placed on other devices to ensure stability during use. Hygiene demands that dildos not be shared with others, or condoms be placed on dildos to prevent the spread of STD's.

Electricity
Using electricity in BDSM play seems a scary notion to most people, but it can easily be made safe provided two simple rules are followed: a) only use devices powered by low-voltage batteries, and certainly no main-powered appliances; and b) avoid placing any contacts above the waist (including hands or arms), as even small currents to the heart or brain can disrupt those organs' delicate electrical activity with serious consequences. Popular devices include "TENS" units designed for the relief of muscle and back pain; and "Violet Wands" which use a radio frequency discharge, and can be used above the waist provided the face is avoided. Any form of this play can be dangerous.

Enforced Chastity
In BDSM / S/m circles, meaning the banning or physically preventing one from achieving orgasm or any form of genital stimulation. A means of domination over one's submissive. A device (lockable) panty-type which when worn prevents any type of genital stimulation.

Exhibitionism
Scening involving the display of public / private exhibitionism in order to exert control and / or humiliation.

Face Slapping
Involves play where a moderate amount of slapping of the face is used for humiliation / control. This play can be dangerous if an eye is struck, etc.

Fisting (Anal / Vaginal)
Play which involves placing or attempting to place the entire hand (or even both hands) in the rectum / vagina. The hand is only formed into a fist, and once fully inserted, requires an extreme gentleness, care, and patience. Involves moving of the fist in and out of the orifice and can be a dangerous technique if not performed correctly. Proper study should be done, before attempting such, and after care is extremely important.

Flogger

A whip device usually with many "tails". Used on buttocks or back, generally to make nerve sensations greater. Floggers can be used on the genital areas. Can be used for play or punishment. This form of play is not for the novice, and can be dangerous.

Flogging horse

A device used to secure one on this bench-like, padded, sawhorse. Usually made waist height, with the use of tethers attached to wall or floor to secure the submissive. A well designed horse will allow open spread usage of the submissive when mounted properly upon.

Forced Masturbation

Scenes where the submissive is forced to perform masturbation in front of/for the Dominant or others as a form of erotic / sensual play or humiliation.

Forced Servitude

A form of play involving the submissive acting as a servant / maid to the Dominant. May be played out in public or in private as a form of humiliation.

Gags

To restrict the use of the mouth by inserting a gag, in various textures (i.e., cloth, leather, ball gag, etc.). When using gags, it is important to remember that these only be worn for short periods of time. This form of play can be **dangerous.**

Golden Shower

Play which involves urinating on one's submissive or vice versa.

Hairbrush Spanking

Play which involves the use of a hairbrush to inflict pain on the buttocks. Commonly used in "naughty boy / girl" scenes for punishment.

Hair Pulling

Pulling of one's hair for the purpose of pain / humiliation. Used often in heavy sceneing.

Hand Jobs
Using the hands to perform sexual gratification on a man's penis. Stroking of the penis to facilitate orgasm.

Humiliation
To humiliate the submissive by requiring them to perform things they normally would not do, most commonly in public (i.e., wearing revealing clothing; having sex in public; playing out puppy, boy / girl scenes, etc.).

Orgasm Control
When one is forced to release or hold their body's desires to orgasm. Can be used in play or punishment.

Pain
In broad terms, pain is the body's warning that something is; however, our pain responses are very complex and it is very easy to produce the effect of pain without doing any real harm to the body. The "pain threshold" at which a stimulus crosses the boundary between intense sensation and pain is a gray area in terms of our perception. BDSM is associated in most people's minds with potentially painful activities, sometimes referred to as "pain games". It is true; however, that some people actually enjoy or at least get some satisfaction out of the intense physical sensation. Some of the satisfaction may be attributed to the release of body chemicals also known as "endorphins". Most player's interests are a mixture of physical aspects and the psychological dynamics of Domination and submission, and some play with hardly any physical pain at all. Those for whom the interest in pain is predominant are sometimes referred to sadists and masochists rather than Dominants and submissives. **After care** is, and monitoring the one receiving pain, is mandatory. Not for the novice for play.

Piercing
Piercing of the body with a thin sharp object such as a needle. There are two types of play, permanent and temporary. Permanent piercing is done with a thicker needle which enables jewelry to be easily inserted. Temporary piercing is done with a smaller, thinner needle which can be removed without permanent scarring after the session is completed. (i.e., nipple piercing, ear piercing, genital piercing). Mostly done to enhance the sensual areas of the skin. Piercing should be done be a professional.

Pony Slave

Scenes involving the submissive being dressed or made up as to portray a "pony". Scenes might include mouth bits, harnesses, saddles, riding crops, etc. Note: Riding your pony can cause serious damage to their backs, hips, joints.

Public Exposure

Play which involves exposing oneself in public (i.e., flashing). Used for control / humiliation purposes.

Pussy Worship

The practice of play involving the "worship" of the female genitalia. Scenes may involve the cleaning, licking, shaving, etc. In general, "worship" is a form of erotic play.

Rack

A table-like device which is fitted with pulling or stretching capabilities. Some racks incorporate pulleys, winches or wheels pulling one in opposing directions. Paddles or whips are generally used on the person on a rack.

Saint Andrews Cross

This is a cross made in an X formation. It is generally angled and self-supporting. Some are suspended from ceilings, or mounted directly to a wall. The cross has leather restraints for arms, legs and body, Some have hooks along the edges for a person to be "laced" to the cross. Used for sexual play, or punishment can be administered while attached to the cross.

Sensory Deprivation

Play which involves "depriving" the submissive of certain sensory perceptions. May include blindfolds, bondage, gags, etc.

Shaving

Using a razor or straight blade to shave hair from the body. **Note:** Shaving of the genital area should be done with extreme care.

Slings

Slings are made in many designs and shapes, but their use is to open access to the genitalia for play or punishment. This form of suspension causes fatigue rather quickly, so after-care should be taken as well as care during such use. Not for the novice.

Spreader Bar

A bar type device used to "spread" apart arms / legs of the submissive. Bars can be made of common, inexpensive materials such as dowel rods, pvc pipe, broomsticks, etc.

Stocks

A type of bondage "furniture" based on the medieval form of stocks used for punishment. Stocks usually consist of two hinged of wood with semi-circular holes which when locked together form a ring large enough for the head / neck and wrists to be placed inside.

Strapping

A length of material, most commonly leather, used for striking the body.

Suspension

An advanced form of bondage in which the whole body is "suspended" off the ground and hanging "free in space". **Note:** not for the novice, use of properly designed equipment is advised.

Tattoo

A permanent form of "marking the submissive" as property.

Table Play

A padded table, where the submissive is restrained for play. The table has many securing points to offer different positions for play or examination. Tables can be used as racks if outfitted accordingly.

Tampon Training

Tampons inserted into the rectum, used as an anal plug, for play or punishment.

Waxing

Using warmed wax as a form of erotic sensation. Common areas of waxing are the buttocks, breast area, back, etc. The process of using hot wax in scening. The wax most commonly used are candles. **Note:** Some types of wax, beeswax for instance, have a tendency to become extremely hot during burning and should always be done carefully to prevent permanent burning/scarring of the skin.

Whipping

A device consisting of a long, flexible striking surface. Whipping the body with a whip type device as a form of punishment.

Whipping Post

Designs vary according to builder, but the principle is to have a tall post with tethers that hang down, to attach a person from their wrists. Used for positioning a submissive for ease of whipping. Some Dominants use the "whipping post" for punishment only, and never for play.

After an intense scene, people can have various reactions anywhere from several hours to a few days. Doms and subs/slaves can experience an emotional response called Top or Sub Drop. Each, in their own way, has reached a level rarely achieved in daily life, and which, very often, neither is prepared for.

Top/Sub drop is the coming down and the return to normality. This can happen quickly or slowly. It can be a nice experience, or a bad one. The effects of sub drop are similar to a kind of depressive state. There can be spontaneous outbursts of emotion, such as tears, irrationality, fear, or any number of other things. They can last almost no time at all, or they can go on for hours. Many subs/slaves like to be held after a scene. Some people can be very emotional after playing and need to be taken care of. It is a good idea to have some snacks and juices and/or caffeinated drinks handy, as well as plenty of water. If you are not a couple/group living together, you should keep in touch. You may not experience a drop, but a follow up call is still a good idea. You will be taking care of an emotional need that can be as strong as the physical need you have already taken care of.

AFTERCARE is usually given to the sub by their Dom/Master. Cuddling and comforting is a great way to wrap things up. Aftercare can also be one of the best parts of a scene. Many couples/partners talk of a level of intimacy and closeness that they don't get otherwise.

Chapter Six

Different Types of BDSM Relationships

Many people that are new to the Lifestyle, or outsiders looking in, think all of BDSM relationships are the same. That there is One Dominant, One sub/slave; the Dominant tells the sub what to do, the sub gets beat just for the heck of it, and that all subs are made to walk around on a collar and leash naked all the time on their hands and knees. While this might be true for some, it is not true for most! Here are some of the most common types of BDSM relationships a couple outside BDSM that are closely related.

There are sexual and non-sexual, service, training, age play, and more. I want to just touch on the most common forms that you will see in real life and cyber.

D/s - Dominant / submissive

This is the most basic and common form you will hear about and encounter in a BDSM relationship. This usually consists of a Dominant (Male or Female) and one or more submissives/slaves. The power exchange or D/s in this type of relationship is not normally practiced in a 24/7 way, meaning that there are large parts of a submissive's life that are not dictated by the Dominant and the sub is free to do, say, wear, act, etc. in any way that he/she wants. D/s is usually practiced in a scene related or training environment, or reserved for specific parts of a sub's life or specific hours. The couple can be partially vanilla at times, can be two or more strangers getting together for a scene, or can be a paid Dominant with a sub. Many times it will include a Dominant that trains certain submissives in certain forms of service for Dominants. There are many exceptions to my definition, but this is the most common form it will take.

M/s - Master(Mistress) / slave

This form of power exchange is a much deeper and stricter version of Dominance and submission. There is a Master/Mistress and either one or more submissives and/or slaves (read previous blog post on sub versus slave to understand the definitions more). Remember that just because it is M/s, does not automatically mean the sub is a slave. You will normally see this type of relationship in a committed couple or committed poly group, cyber or real life. The origins are based in real life 24/7 situations, where the sub/slave lives with her/his Master/Mistress. The Master/Mistress will have rules and guidelines that dictate how the sub/slave is to act, dress, interact with others, etc... in most parts of the sub/slave's life. This relationship always includes tasks and punishments as well. There are many people that are in online relationships that say they are in M/s vs D/s based relationships. The longer you are in the Lifestyle, you will learn that most real life BDSM'ers do not recognize online as a real form of M/s. I think it can be if both participants are open, honest with the other one.

S&M – Sadomasochism
In its purest form, this involves two people, one known as a Sadist that likes to inflict sexual pain, and a Masochist, one that likes to receive sexual pain. There are many people in and around BDSM that are purely Sadomasochists. They do not describe or see themselves as Dominants or submissives. They are in BDSM simply for the sexual gratification of whips, chains, clamps, bondage, wax play, etc. Now, D/s and M/s can certainly involve S&M, but does not necessarily mean it has to. There are many couples that like to have what is considered normal sex without ropes, chains, floggers or toys, but practice the D/s or M/s lifestyle.

Taken-in-Hand Relationships
A Taken In Hand relationship is a fully-committed wholehearted sexually-exclusive marriage in which the husband is firmly and actively in charge and he puts his wife and their relationship first.

It is a consciously and consensually male controlled, sexually exclusive, relationship in which the man's power is real and for the purpose of cultivating a deeply connected, fully engaged relationship. How the man expresses his dominance is an individual matter, but it's for the benefit of the relationship rather than being purely self-serving. The man protects and cherishes the woman he leads. The woman responds positively to her man's control.

The wives in Taken In Hand relationships tend not to claim to be submissive (though their husbands may well consider them to be so) and strongly prefer not to be the one in charge in their relationship. They do respect, honor, obey and appreciate their husbands and strive to please them.

The husbands in Taken In Hand relationships tend not to claim to be dominant but prefer to be the one wearing the pants in their marriage. They do enjoy dominating and submitting their wife when necessary to maintain their position.

Now, remember, just because I have given you what I define as the most common types of relationships, does not mean that there isn't cross over, combinations, and exceptions to every one I have named. There are also more that I have not mentioned because there are just too many. I hope this helps you in your quest and furthers your own path on the journey.

Building Foundations of D/s Relationship

There are many people out there that either do not like the S&M of BDSM, or just don't practice it. These relationships could be called simple D/s or a Taken In Hand type of relationship.

I'm not drawing a distinction between 24/7 D/s and M/s relationships, because I find that different people use the terms interchangeably. I'm talking about relationships that involve a full-time power exchange. For me, that means relationships in which the two (or more) people involved always relate to one another from a power-based dynamic, and that this dynamic extends outside the time that the people spend in one another's presence.

There is a distinction between fantasy and reality. 24/7 relationships happen when you're doing it for reasons beyond orgasm (even if arousal and orgasm are a big, or even essential, part of the draw). This is not a huge ongoing role-play scenario. It's an intensification of the power-based parameters in which you live your everyday life. If you simply try to extend a role-play scenario into your entire relationship, you'll find that the narrow parameters of a persona or character are simply not big enough to encompass who you are, and need to be, every hour of every day.

24/7 is not about restricting yourself to a specific set of characteristics the way you can for an hour or two in a scene. It's about bringing all of who you are to the table and offering it within a full-spectrum relationship. That means you're doing it regardless of what you're wearing (leather, work drag, bunny slippers…) and where you are (bedroom, dungeon, airport, family dinner) and what you're doing (having sex, working, eating breakfast, hanging out with friends). Yes, this means you may need to find ways to scale up and down the overt visibility of your relationship. No, it does not mean you're turning it on or off at will. A lot of the classic "it's just play" concepts that you might hear in a BDSM 101 workshop are going to go right out the window here because what you are doing is not a scene. It comes with a whole different – related, but different – psychology.

Being in a hurry has probably brought on more heartaches than any single thing we hear about when discussing failed relationships. Those submissive urges can be very strong and sometimes overpower common sense unless you really keep things from getting out of hand. Without first building a foundation of love, trust and respect, there isn't much hope of any relationship succeeding, especially a D/s one. Searching for the Dominant of your dreams is pretty much like dating in the vanilla world but with an added twist. You will have to trust this person with your life and well-being. You have to really know this person and I personally do not believe this can happen before you have had several months on which to base your judgment. Don't be afraid to ask for references from people he/she knows in the lifestyle. If this creates a problem because you did ask, I'd consider the possibility that this person has something to hide.

Not fully understanding your limits and the things expected in this lifestyle can lead to some serious problems that can be easily avoided. Learn all you can about D/s and yourself. Make checklist of activities with your potential dominant and find out what things do and do not interest you. You have the right and obligation to honestly express your feelings on activities within this lifestyle. No one likes or needs them all and keeping your real feelings hidden will only lead to problems later. Keep in mind that dominants have limits too. For a relationship to be satisfying and healthy, it has to be based on mutual interests and goals.

Communicating effectively is more than just talking. You have to be able to voice your concerns, hopes, needs, dreams, disappointments, and hurts as well as all the positive emotions you so willingly share. Remember it's also listening to what is said and the way it's said. Gestures, facial expressions and body language often say more than words. Learning some better communication skills is always a good investment for your future. A great deal of the dynamics of a D/s relationship hinges on you openly sharing your fantasies and fears. If there is something that's causing you to be anxious or has left you unfulfilled, it's your duty to communicate this to your dominant. The same applies for the things that have given you pleasure or satisfaction. You have to share what's happening inside that submissive head and heart. Remember, even the best dominant is not a mind reader.

Intense power relationships will bring you face to face with whatever issues you need to work on. Your ability to sustain your D/s relationship depends on you and your partner's willingness to deal with them, and your mutual willingness to deal with theirs. Hint: if the same thing keeps going wrong in every relationship, you don't just need to find the right person; you need to change yourself. At the same time as you both commit to working on yourselves, you also need to find a way to balance this with a commitment to accepting each other as you are. While you can work on specific things, and while major change does take place sometimes, you cannot fundamentally change a person into something they are not, and you certainly can't expect major change to happen quickly or exactly as you'd like it to. So don't enter into a 24/7 relationship if your happiness is going to be dependent on a radical or immediate personality shift on the others' part.

D/s relationships are intense. Have I mentioned that? They are intense, soul-searching relationships that affect every moment of every day. The kind of exploration and self-revelation that so often comes with D/s can make you go a bit nuts if you have no outside support. That support can take many forms:

Participation in a kink community can be incredibly helpful—it can provide relationship models for you to look at and learn from or discard as needed. Even if everyone around you does their kink differently than you do, that can help you better understand who you are (and are not) and what you're doing (and not doing).

Reading, workshops, discussion groups, and any number of other educational resources can similarly give you ideas to chew on, frameworks that may or may not work for you, and language to help you understand and express what you're getting up to.

And last but not least, friends you can talk to about D/s. Non-kinky (but kink-friendly) friends are a great start, because the kind of challenges that come up in D/s are often similar to those in any other relationship. But frequently enough, D/s relationship issues will also have a character all their own, and even the most open-minded or well-intentioned vanilla friend may have a hard time truly getting it. It can be extremely helpful to build friendships with fellow D/s practitioners so you can offer each other a supportive shoulder when needed. Hint: Don't wait until you need help… start building those friendships right away, and make sure you offer your own listening ear.

A brief caution: a classic warning sign that a D/s relationship is not so healthy is when one of the partners tells the other not to talk about it with anyone else, or not to participate in community. Of course you want to maintain basic respect for each other and your relationship – airing your dirty laundry for all to see, or trashing your partner loudly at a play party, is just not classy. But having one or two trusted friends to turn to in times of trouble can be essential and a wise dominant will encourage the submissive to seek out support rather than discouraging it.

Patience takes a long time to build in great depth, and often is the Dominant's job is to hold back, not to rush forward. Taking on responsibility for another human being in a polarized power situation is simply not something that's wise to do quickly or carelessly. Take your time. Learn what you need to learn about yourself, about them, about how to do this well and feel good about it. Don't extend past your own limits because you feel pressure to do it all right-now-tout-de-suite. I do say that it's often the dominant's job to hold back, because sometimes a submissive can be gung-ho and champing at the bit while their dominant is feeling overwhelmed and struggling to hold tight.

Lastly, it takes continued work, communication, and an open willingness to continuously adapt to make a long lasting and loving D/s relationship work and grow stronger. We choose to be open to everyone about the fact we live a 24/7 BDSM or D/s lifestyle. It makes it much easier on us. Many of our vanilla friends do not understand and others have simply stopped talking to us. We are ok with that. Because for us, we are most happy being ourselves and being open with who we are. But, it is up to you and your partner to determine how much you let your vanilla friends know.

Living a D/s Relationship 24/7

D/s is possible 24/7. It takes work and patience, trust, open communication and knowing each other very well. I am a slave and I always remember my status and place. In any situation, I always think about how Padrone would guide me. Padrone never forgets his responsibilities in having a slave

The life as a 24/7 slave is what I have always wanted. It is a part of my very nature, to serve and please my Padrone. For Him to have very strict control on me shows I am very loved and cared for. With all of the rules in place and restrictions I have, Padrone does that very well.

Living in a D/s relationship is extremely interesting and at times very challenging. You really do have to change your whole way of thinking, and of how you look at life. When I first began talking to Padrone, I didn't think that I would end up being collared by Him, let alone become His life partner and move in with Him as His slave. However, as time went on, it became obvious to us both, that what we have is something rare and special, and though it may not be everyone's idea of paradise, for us, it is a winning combination.

A lot of people in the Lifestyle may think that living in a 24/7 would be the ultimate, and for me it is. But, there are many speed bumps to be negotiated along the way. The simple act of living together is difficult enough in a vanilla relationship, but when the relationship is D/s, it brings a whole new set of conditions to adjust to. For example, in a vanilla relationship, the decision about where things are put becomes a joint one - a discussion between two people about what looks or works best. In our relationship, Padrone decides what goes where. I can, and do, respectfully suggest things, and sometimes my suggestions are taken up, but in the end, the final say is Padrone's.

The way I look at my life is very different now. Getting my head around some things has taken time, but I am secure and confident and know exactly who and what I am, and I am totally comfortable with it. At home, things are very relaxed and we do normal things like laugh and joke around, or watch TV. The basis for our relationship is D/s and no matter what situation we are in, I never, ever forget that He is Padrone and I am slave. There is a lot more D/s going on than most people would realize. A glance, a certain tone in His voice, a certain movement or a simple request for a cup of coffee may all seem like normal things, but the way it's done leaves no doubt in my mind just who is in control.

I believe there is difference between D/s and BDSM. D/s is the show or feel of Dominance and submission. There is service and outward respect and obedience shown. The BDSM part to me is the bondage, the playing, the pain, the S&M. The D/s is constant. The Dominance and submission is evident in our relationship, but in a way that is unobtrusive. The D/s part can be shown without lots of people thinking much of it or noticing it. Some examples would be in the way I always walk slightly behind Padrone or that he always leads me by my hand whenever we are in public.

We do have our disagreements every once in a while, just like any other relationship, but the boundaries are more clearly defined and there is a more consistent feeling all the time. I am secure in the knowledge that Padrone loves me, that I am owned by Him, and I know that fact will never change or waiver no matter what happens.

So does what we have, make our relationship a 24/7 D/s one? I feel that it is and I know that Padrone does too. There is no time when I feel that I am not His and that is reflected in my acceptance of His collar and he in accepting me as His. I do not think that a 24/7 D/s relationship must reflect one which represents level 9 of submission. I personal do not feel that that is possible. However, I do feel that the level to which we have taken our relationship is possible to maintain every day.

So, whether you choose to label your relationship as a D/s, M/s, or simple BDSM one, it can be maintained 24/7 to a certain degree at all times.

Can Love Exist in a BDSM Relationship?

Can love exist in a BDSM relationship, or is it just two people satisfying mutual needs and gaining gratification? Is it Love a sub feels for her Dom or is it 'Dom worship'? Does the Dom really care for His sub or does He just have a more fond feeling and a sense of responsibility for her?

Whether or not love should enter into a dominant / submissive relationship is something that is debated within the BDSM community. Whereas most will agree that there should be some form of caring involved, actually falling in love is often frowned upon. In the kinky world, things are a bit more complicated when it comes to relationship dynamics. There are fewer expectations, I think, of well-defined romantic relationships, than in the non-kinky world. With all the different personal preferences, there are more options than ever.

Those who frown on falling in love would argue that when such intense emotions enter into a BDSM relationship, they can interfere with the Dominant / submissive aspect of the relationship. When a submissive is in love with her Master, she is more prone to feelings of jealousy. She is also more prone to desire all of the things that one associates with falling in love, such as romance, marriage and family. When a Dominant falls in love with his submissive, he may be less likely to subject her to the humiliation, pain and control that he would normally offer to a submissive.

Those who say that falling in love is good in a Dominant / submissive relationship believe that such strong emotions serve to enhance the relationship. They believe that a Dominant who is in love with his submissive will be mindful of his submissive's safety in a way he might not be otherwise. It is also believed that a submissive who is in love with her Dominant will be more serious about the relationship and less prone to play games. She will be more obedient and will put the needs of her dominant first in a way she might not do otherwise.

There are many people I know who are part of different BDSM dynamics, and don't have romantic relationships with their partners. In my view, love is very important as part of a long-term relationship such vulnerability on a deep level. For me, being with someone as a slave has to include love. However, that's not always the case. There are several instances where love has nothing to do with it. There are connections such as friendship, service and desire.

Some relationships are sexual, without being more connected than just washing the back of someone who washed yours. Many choose this option when their primary partner (often a marriage partner) is unaware of or unwilling to participate in their kinky desires. This can often lead to cheating, and though non-monogamy is actually approved of in the kink world, dishonesty tends to be frowned upon.

Friendship can also be the basis for a BDSM based relationship. Those who might not want to be sexually involved, or who might want sex and kink but already have a romantic partner with no desire for another, can choose to not get romantically involved with someone. There are people who are married to vanilla partners and are deeply in love with them, but fulfill their kinky needs with others. Though they do that, some have no room, romantically, to love another in that romantic way. Still others cannot see being in love with someone who they might cause pain for, or dominate, or submit to (on the other end of that stick). It's a choice to separate the two kinds of relationships, and for some it works well.

When embarking on a Dominant / submissive relationship, it is important to decide ahead of time what your boundaries are and communicate them to your partner. Nobody knows ahead of time if they will end up falling in love, but it is important to talk about how you will deal with it if it happens. What if one of you falls in love and the other one doesn't? This seems to be where the biggest problem can be, because the desires of one change whereas the desires of the other remains the same.

Open communication is the key to having a good relationship with your partner. Whether you believe it is a good idea or not to fall in love with your dominant or submissive...communication with one another will help you deal with the issue.

Jealousy in a D/S Relationship

Becoming a true submissive is a process. Even if you feel you were born to serve a dominant, there are going to be areas that are going to be very difficult at times. One of these areas is in regard to jealousy. When you give yourself to a dominant, you are telling him that you belong to him and that you are entrusting him with your well-being... physically, mentally, and emotionally. Although this sounds incredibly romantic, it can also be very difficult. It means you must, at times, sacrifice your wants and needs for the wants and needs of your dominant.

Jealousy is a negative emotion and can cause a great deal of trouble in a relationship. Jealousy can rip a relationship apart if it gets out of control and may cause you to lose your partner. Losing them is the very thing we are most afraid of when we are jealous, is it not?

You have the right to feel jealous. How you express that emotion is another matter. You don't have the right to control another's actions with jealousy. Do not attack your partner out of jealousy. Express your feelings in a positive manner.

A good dominant/submissive relationship is one in which there is a lot of communication. Much of this communication should take place before you actually make any kind of commitment to the relationship. There are certain rules that should be established ahead of time. Whereas some dominants are happy with one submissive, there are others who desire more than one submissive. This is something you should discuss with your dominant ahead of time, especially if you are prone to jealousy.

Jealousy might seem like a sign of love. But when someone uses it to try to control what you do, this isn't love or submission - it's control. Everyone has the right to talk to anyone they want to. It also isn't in keeping with the tradition of being a submissive to use jealousy to control another's actions.

Jealousy, in and of itself, is not wrong. Jealousy is a natural emotion. What causes the problem is how we act upon the jealousy that we are feeling. Jealousy can cause people to act out in very unbecoming ways. For a submissive, such acting out can mean the end of the relationship with her dominant.

No one should purposely provoke jealousy in a partner. That is a dangerous game to play. It is the Doms job to create an atmosphere of safety for his submissive and a submissive should never provoke jealousy in her Dom as it is her job to demonstrate that she is loyal and cannot be had by another who happens along.

Giving yourself to a dominant means trusting him to always keep you safe and to keep your well-being in mind. This doesn't mean you will always agree with him. This doesn't mean you will always enjoy certain things. What it does mean is that as long as you are committed to the relationship, you will trust him and the decisions that he makes.

As long as you are consumed by the negative energy of jealousy, it is unlikely that any positive resolution will be possible. You must let go of your own suffering, step back and examine the relationship in depth, and then make a reasoned response. Only once the emotion has been defused, can clear thinking become possible.

Never be afraid to ask your dominant questions...especially in the beginning. It can be very easy to overlook certain warning signs if you are very taken in by a dominant's many attributes. If you do care for your relationship and want to keep the relationship on track and moving in a positive direction, then use a NAME statement to address the behavior.

The NAME statement shows respect for your partner and is very specific. This kind of communication puts the emphasis on what you see and what you feel, not on blame toward your partner.

N - name the specific behavior that you find causes you to feel jealous

A - announce the specific setting … time & place the behavior occurred

M - mention your reaction & the feeling it arouses in you

E - explain and own your feelings

Most of all, always be open and honest with your partner and keep the lines of communication open.

Chapter Seven

Dominant's Role

This section applies to Real Life and Cyber Domination

Being Dominant is a state of mind. It is not a sex act, it is not a game, and it is not a role. It is a state of being and is totally asexual (neither male nor female). First and foremost, a Dominant is always a Gentleman or Lady. There is no excuse for being impolite or rude to others. Save this for the submissive that needs and requires this of their Dominant.

Self-control, knowledge, and a questioning mind, along with the ability to listen, understand, and question, are the foundations on which a Dominant personality should be built. Next is the ability to accept responsibility. A Dominant should understand that in a Dominant submissive (D/s) relationship, the submissive is going to place their faith in the Dom in many ways. It is inherent in a Dominant submissive (D/s) relationship that the submissive needs to give up some level of control and responsibility to the Dominant. Acceptance of that control must sit comfortably with the Dominant. To have another hand over control of their life, (or at least parts of it) to you is an awesome feeling. It must be borne with great care, and never abused. So, a Dominant does not abuse the power they are given. They never take that power, they are given it out of love, trust, and respect, and the feeling that they can improve the quality of another's life.

Along with responsibility, the Dominant must have patience. Patience in a Dominant is a requisite too, because there may be many times when a submissive may not reach expectations. This may not be due to any failing on the submissive's part, and so the Dominant must show patience, and a calming influence: an ability to help the sub, to achieve what they both want, in a structured and sensible way, and never to criticize when things don't go well.

Being single-minded in what they want is another Dominant. The ability to have a vision, and through whatever gets in the way, to be able to preserve that in their mind, and make progress towards that goal, irrespective of what it might be, is likely to be another characteristic seen in most Dominants. Through all these there also remains the fact, that someone who is able to accept the responsibility for another, make informed decisions about life altering processes, of having an ability to manage, and accept change, and alter the plan to suit prevailing circumstances. One's care for another must by definition take their hopes, fears, needs, and desires into account; these needs will change over time, and so, as they do, the original vision that one may have had for a relationship may well have to change. The inability to see that is not conducive to Dominance.

A Dominant must always be in control. Drugs, even alcohol, are mind and body controlling agents. They affect relationships and most importantly can affect a scene, therefore taking away the control the Dominant MUST have.

A Dominant is always honest. To lie is to show You cannot be trusted and a sub/slave must be able to trust You to respect you. Every sub/slave knows that not every Dominant is super experienced and will respect You much more if You tell the truth. Be honest with a sub/slave about Your level of experience with others. They can even help You to gain experience, which can be an enjoyable learning process. Tell them up-front if You do not wish a monogamous relationship. Most submissives understand and even expect this in a Dominant. You may not get "that" sub/slave, but You will not lose her/his respect.

A Dominant expects, but does not demand respect. No Dominant demands strangers to call him/her Master/Mistress. Respect is earned over time. Demanding Master/Mistress on Your name means nothing and is a word that when not earned, is meaningless and makes You appear to be petty and childish. Those that know and respect You will call you Master or Mistress when You earn it, not before. Remember, to other Dominants, You are not Their Master/Mistress. You are Their equal. Do not demand Them too ever call You that.

A Dominant knows and understands the differences between needs, desires and wants. The sub/slave may want a 24/7 relationship with an understanding Dominant. Even in a Master/slave relationship, the Dominant must always know if the sub/slave needs a little softer or harder touch.

The Dominant must be flexible to be a true Master. Remember, even subs/slaves have feelings.

It is the duty of a Dominant to remember that submission is a gift. To misuse this gift is abusive. When the sub/slave is not free to take back the gift, it is no longer a gift.

A Dominant must take only the amount of subs/slaves they can properly handle, control, love, comfort and care for.

A Dominant should only take a submissive that will match Him/Her. A sub/slave that is not into whips should not belong to a Dominant that loves to whip submissives.

After-care by Dominant after a scene is essential to ensure the sub/slave is emotionally stable. During a scene, they are filled with hormones. Afterwards, the body reduces them and may cause severe depression to the extent of being suicidal. The submissive must be made to understand the depression and or emotional release is normal and expected. Normal emotions will return in hours to a day. Anything longer is a sign of emotional instability in the sub/slave and must be corrected before doing another scene.

A Dominant HAS to know and understand what the needs, desires and wants of a sub/slave are. Failure to do so may harm the submissive emotionally and mentally.

Dishonorable Acts

- To allow a sub/slave to be actually harmed in ANY way.
- To allow a sub/slave's rights to be violated.
- To play with and discard a sub/slave just for amusement (exception is a submissive that has declared this is the treatment they need).
- Unless the sub/slave has declared themselves to be unowned, another Dominant's interference in a relationship.
- To chase after or scene with Another's sub/slave without the other Dominant's permission and full knowledge.

Dominant's Suggested Guideline for subs/slave Protocols

- Have them wear slave bells. The constant soft jingling of the bells is soothing and a certain reminder of their submission.
- When the sub/slave has broken a rule, talk to them as You punish....and make them speak in detail about why, whatever they did, was wrong.
- Make the sub/slave take their clothes off every day as soon as they enter Your house.
- A beautiful, special collar will make any sub/slave joyous. Take the time to select the right one, and have them wear it as often as possible.
- Have them call You each day at a specified time, no excuses.
- Whenever possible, have the sub/slave kneel before You and ask to sit beside You on the furniture.
- Choose the sub/slave's hairstyle and go with them to get it cut to Your specifications.
- Whenever possible, have them display themselves whenever You come into the room.....legs spread, shirt unbuttoned. No matter what position You take, they have to be sure Your view is unobstructed
- When around the kids or vanilla friends/family, make sure the sub/slave has an alternative title for You besides Master.....such as "my Love" etc.
- Use them sexually in a rough, selfish way when You feel like it....interrupting whatever they were doing.
- Have them crawl to bed each night.
- Choose their clothing each day.
- Have the sub/slave get Your daily wardrobe ready for You the night before....laid out, ironed etc.
- After punishment, have them kiss Your feet and thank You for loving them enough to correct them.
- Have them bring a warm towel and wash and massage Your feet each day after work.
- Get them tattooed if it is a permanent relationship with Your choice of what and where.
- Respect, but push their limits.
- Ask them each night what they did that day that You would not have approved of. This gets them in the habit of being completely honest, and also makes them conscious of the things they could do better each day.

- Teach them exactly how You want them to kneel, and demand perfection.
- Reward your sub/slave by allowing them to please You sexually.
- Supervise their workout routine. Make sure that if you implement this, your sub/slave is capable of keeping up with whatever workout you choose. You do not want to hurt them.
- Have them polish Your boots weekly, on their knees, at Your feet.
- Negotiate until you are both comfortable with the terms and limits set and then sign a contract.
- Teach them to always ask You first if you would like something to eat or drink, before preparing something for themselves.
- Some evenings, keep them on a leash and take them with You no matter what You do....even if You do not speak to or include them in Your activities.
- When appropriate, they are only to speak when spoken to.
- Reward your sub/slave by giving them delicious pleasure.
- When it suits You, instruct them not to make eye contact with You without Your command.
- Have them keep their body hygiene as you instructed them initially, at all times.
- Conduct random inspections of their body to make sure they keep to Your specifications.
- Make them wear a butt-plug under their clothes when they go out alone.
- For transgressions, make sure You follow up with punishment swiftly and precisely, then forget and forgive.
- Master the art of the meaningful piercing stare.
- Give them reading assignments to further their education in BDSM or the erotic arts.
- Test them on the reading assignments, to make sure they learned the appropriate lessons from each one.
- Make it their responsibility to put away toys after play and punishment, and to keep them clean and neat.
- Call them Your slut, Your pet, etc.
- Have them make a list of the 10 things that make them the most self-conscious, uncomfortable or embarrassed.
- Work with them on the list (if possible), so that they conquer those fears and hesitations.
- Sometimes, pamper them.....wash their body and hair, having them remain perfectly still as You turn and move them about.

- Hand feed them on occasion.
- Praise their dedication when they have pleased You well.
- Instruct them that they may never touch Your body without permission.
- Make a rule, when possible, no clothing in the house.
- As a punishment deny their orgasm. Make sure that You cum but they do not.
- Have them wear nipple clamps under clothing out to dinner.
- On Your birthday, let them receive Your spankings.
- Spend time training them how to move gracefully to please You.
- Another form of punishment is to stand them in the corner, bare assed for a period of time.
- Pet them often and praise them when they have done well.
- Whenever possible, have them sleep in a cage.
- Buy clothes to Your liking.
- Teach them things....expand their knowledge.....in a patient Fatherly way.
- When You travel, call and have them masturbate for You.
- If You choose to play with others, make sure Your slave knows who is first in Your heart.....and that some things are just for them.
- When outside together, lead them by the hand and have them walk beside or slightly behind you.
- Have them wake you with a routine (coffee, kisses, singing etc).
- Teach them patience.
- Videotape Your sessions and watch them together.
- When you feel the need to pamper them, hand feed them and have them feed You.
- Keep a list of their transgressions in a little book....let them slip for a while...thinking You are not noticing.....then one day, bring out the book and have a day of atonement.
- Have them wear a collar 24/7, even to work if its possible. Make sure to pick a collar that looks like a choker or necklace, but one that will always remind them of who they are.
- Have them take sexy pictures of themselves and email them to You when You are at work.
- Remember to kiss and caress away their tears.
- Make sure that they always know You love them, during punishment and pleasure.
- Have them fall asleep with Your cock in their mouth.
- Remind them always that Your word is law.

- Make sure that your slave is and feels safe at all times (when with You and when You are apart)
- Be consistent.
- Take the time to talk to them and learn their fears, dreams, and fantasies. Use the knowledge You gain.

Chapter Eight

The submissive/slave Role

Submission is an action of personal strength. To overcome internal resistance, the submissive must control their desire or need to maintain personal control in the creation and delivery of all personal decisions. It is defined as the trait to willingly yield to the will of another person or a superior force.

In the vast world of BDSM, there are many variations of relationships, but also types of submissives. Most people say you cannot classify submissives because they fall into more than one category. This is true. There are many shades of grey in between (pun intended). Everyone submits differently, depending on their own personality, relationship dynamic, and view of submission.

A submissive is a person who gives up control and gets emotional or sexual satisfaction from aspects of submission which may include serving or being used by the Dominant. A submissive usually only submits during a scene, during sex, or during certain well defined and set parameters. They may or may not follow rules or protocols outside of the above situations. At all other times, they are on equal footing with their Dominant. These people also normally don't give their Dominant the title of Master.

A slave is an individual who is wholly under the control and power of a Master. A slave is the property of their Master. They freely surrendered their rights and privileges as an individual. They thrive on the opportunity to provide unconditional service and to exceed their Owner's expectations. A person that identifies themselves as a slave usually feels happy by making their Owner happy. They feel down and depressed if they perform a task incorrectly or make their Owner angry. Slaves normally live in a 24/7 TPE (total power exchange) relationship with their Masters.

Now, having defined the differences between the two, are there exceptions? Well of course there are. The above definitions are what is generally accepted by the BDSM community at large. With the explosion of BDSM on the internet, there are many variations to both defined roles. There are now cyber slaves, cyber submissives, and many roles in between that have not yet been defined.

There are those that think defining themselves as a slave, means they are more devoted or more submissive. I don't agree. You can call yourself whatever you want, but your actions and words more clearly define the type of submissive you are.

Is there a difference between a slave and a doormat submissive? Oh yes. A 'doormat' type submissive is a person that does not have any self-esteem at all and feels like they are not worth the slime on the bottom of a dumpster. Their self-image is so low, they usually do anything and everything their Dominant tells them and never complain, no matter how bad the Dominant might be to them. They feel they deserve the roughest and most abusive treatment their Dominant can give, even if such treatment is not warranted. They never ask why because they do not feel they deserve an answer.

A slave usually has very good self-esteem. They know they are prized by their Masters because of the gift of their submission. They have their own convictions and can think for themselves. They do take abuse, but only when it is warranted, as in punishment for something not done correctly or misbehaving. They are strong and loyal, but feel happiest and complete when owned by their 'perfect' Master. They are completed when able to be in total submission 24/7. They love having strict rules and boundaries and always follow them religiously.

Submissives might have some rules but most of them are not that restricting. Cyber submissives and slaves usually have certain protocols they follow, such as emailing the dominant first thing in the morning about their schedules and last thing at night to tell them how their day went.

Does the title of submissive mean you are a stronger person than one that considers themselves to be a slave? Or does a slave mean they are more submissive? They answer according to me is NO to all of the above.

As I stated before, and deeply believe the more I have read, learned, and experienced over the past 20 years, titles do not matter. It is all about what you feel naturally, what you are compelled by your very nature to do or be, that is a true submissive. No matter how far you feel you need to submit, as long as you follow your instincts and your nature, not try to force yourself to submit further than you think you can, you are all equals.

Chapter Nine

General Guide Rules for a sub/slave

- Above all else, the primary focus is to please your Master, whether you are in His presence or not. He knows what is best for you.
- Worship your Master.
- Worship your Master's body.
- The power of your Master's will, thoughts of Him or the hearing of His voice, gives you strength.
- To receive pleasure, you must earn it.
- Trust your Master: His responsibilities, His skills, His hunger and needs, and His concern for your safety, as well as your emotional, psychological, social, sexual, and physical health.
- You are an object of great value - an instrument Master will use to draw out His pleasures.
- You will ask your Master for permission to satisfy whatever need you have before acting on it.
- Your body and mind are the property of your Master.
- Always give thanks to your Master for all you are given, immediately after receiving whatever He has given you, for such things are gifts or privileges granted to you by Him.
- You must be both specific and explicit in your speech.
- Never hesitate when responding to your Master. Your complete focus is important to your continued growth.
- Thank your Master for the discipline and punishments you receive, repeating the reason you were punished.
- You are always submissive to your Master whether He is present or not, ready to please Him at anytime, in any place, under any circumstances, regardless of who may be present. Trust your Master to keep you safe.
- All choices shall be based upon whether or not they will please Master.

- When you are not in the presence of Master and have choices to make, always stay within the boundaries and guidance He has allowed when making decisions.
- Wear the collar of your Master with pride, for it signifies His ownership of you and your devotion to Him.
- Worship your Master's cock when given the opportunity, whether it is hard or soft, for pleasing Him and making Him happy is the main goal. It will make you feel good to do so.
- Your greatest satisfaction is realized when you know you have pleased your Master.
- There can be no greater pain or suffering you will feel then when Master is not pleased with you. Naturally, you may feel depressed, saddened, empty, and lost. Hope He will show His mercy and provide the guidance you will need to be put back on track and be forgiven.
- Your submission should be a natural internal feeling. It is a very powerful force inside you that only a respectable and knowledgeable Master can recognize, control and manage. He understands how your nature influences your behavior. He, too, manages and controls His own naturally dominate state, through sharing a power exchange between you, bonding you tightly to Him.
- Fear nothing, for your Master is always with you and will take care of you.
- Never hesitate in your obedience to your Master.
- Choose to willingly be treated as your Master's property - as long as such treatment is safe and legal.
- When Master feels you are ready and your relationship has progressed to a lifelong commitment, be prepared to receive His unique and permanent mark of ownership upon your body, in a place of His choosing, whether it be a piercing, a tattoo or a branding.
- Remember you are your Master's greatest treasure.
- Learn all the positions Master wants to teach you to the best of your abilities and be prepared to take such positions when required.
- Confess everything to your Master, even when you have been naughty, so that He may decide if such violations require discipline or punishment. Accept whatever decisions He makes by thanking Him for His choice. Focus on how sorry you are for not behaving in the way in which you were taught and for the defilement you brought to yourself and to Him with the unacceptable act which has displeased Him.

- You are a slave - of worth and value to any Master who would find you useful. Your role has been clearly defined by your true nature, enhanced through the teachings of your Master, and will be practiced everyday to the continued pleasure of your Master.
- You have much to learn in order to become a well-trained and well-behaved slave.
- Endure whatever discipline or punishment Master gives you in order to become a better slave for Him.
- Never think of yourself as a weak person, because it takes a strong one to commit to the drive inside yourself, to serve, to obey and to please a Master.
- Strive to continue to be a devoted slave, of good rapport to a Master who truly understands your needs in relationship to His own.
- Give all that you are to a Master in order to become free.
- Never show disrespect towards your Master in any way - no matter where you are - in his presence or not.
- Only in complete submission can you realize the depth of the love you have for Him, your Master.
- Always be attentive to the needs of your Master and always be ready to respond to them to the best of your abilities in whatever way you have developed for Him.
- You are allowed to suggest ways to further your training or use by verbally addressing them your Master when the timing is right.
- Always respond fully, both physically and verbally, to whatever Master does with you. Emotional and physical responses are important to Him. Never hold back any part of your display, regardless of how intense they may be, unless restricted to do so.
- You are a sexual and sensual being.
- Never be passive in serving your Master. Aggressively participate in your exchange with Him.

Chapter Ten

Sub/slave Protocols

At home with no one else present:

- sub/slave should always remove clothing as soon as she/he gets home, unless Master/ Mistress has laid out clothing for the slave or submissive to wear.
- sub/slave should fold clothes neatly or place them in the laundry whenever he/ she gets undressed.
- The sub/slave is to kneel in present posture whenever the Master/ Mistress is due to arrive and wait quietly.
- Whenever the Master/ Mistress is present in a room, the slave must ask permission to enter
- The sub/slave will kneel in the room until the Master/ Mistress gives permission that he or she may move or proceed with cleaning.
- The sub/slave will wear and gratefully accept any toys the Master/ Mistress chooses to insert or adorn her or him with while cleaning or in any other circumstance.
- The sub/slave will not speak unless spoken to and may request an opportunity to speak if there is something pressing to discuss during those periods of time when the Master/ Mistress commands silence.
- The sub/slave may request an opportunity to serve the Dominant
- The sub/slave will always thank the Master/ Mistress for an opportunity to serve whether it was doing a chore or being flogged.
- The sub/slave will keep their eyes averted unless it is the wish of the Master/ Mistress to have their sub/slave look them in the eyes.
- The sub/slave will address the Master/ Mistress not by their first name, but by the title preferred by that Dominant.

In public/ At home with others present:

- A sub/slave will receive visitors at the door with whatever clothing the Master or Mistress commanded.
- A sub/slave will greet visitors in whatever way the Master/ Mistress commands - this may include just taking coats and putting them away, kissing the hand of the guest or kneeling in front of them.
- A sub/slave will not refer to anyone using his or her first name. A sub/slave will use the title Sir or Ma'am combined with their name to differentiate and to make sure that he or she remembers her or his place.
- A sub/slave will serve every person with food and drinks as requested, kneeling to each as the food or drinks are presented.
- A sub/slave will not use furniture and will kneel on the floor until her or his services are required.
- A sub/slave will not speak unless spoken to.
- A sub/slave will remain attentive to make sure that no one has to ask for additional food or drink. A sub/slave should be ready before the command is issued.
- A sub/slave must use high protocol when commanded to do so. This means that the slave will not use first person language when referring to him or herself and will address everyone present with the honorific given to those free.

Sexual Service:

- The sub/slave must be available for sexual service whenever the Dominant requires it. **NOTE:** Some Dominants will keep their sub/slaves to themselves while many others will allow the sub/slave to be shared by any Top that wants them. Make sure that you and your Dominant are clear before you go into this situation about both your preferences.
- The sub/slave must always be ready for any form of sexual service, meaning that her or his body must be prepared in order to make it easy for the Dominant to use him or her.
- The sub/slave will not be allowed to have an orgasm without permission.

- The sub/slave will shave any body hair and maintain this at all times. Failure to do so will result in punishment.
- The sub/slave will be clean and pleasant to all the senses at all times.
- The sub/slave is not allowed to touch her or his Owner's property without permission in any sexual way.

These are but a few of the requirements that some sub/slaves live by. The list is extensive and could be lengthened quite easily. It is always a good idea to have requirements regarding online privileges and privacy, interaction with others not in the lifestyle, as well as people of the opposite sex. In the end, it is the decision of the Dominant what this list should include.

Chapter Eleven

Punishment/ Discipline:

I have been asked by many about different ways to punish unruly or misbehaving subs, when a Dominant should punish their sub and when they should be lenient. Every BDSM relationship is different, so remember, thoughts on punishments different greatly from couple to couple. Culture, age, and personality all play into the way people see punishment. Below is a mixture of my view on punishment as well as a generalization of what I have read on other blogs and in books about their feelings on the subject.

My Padrone and I have the same thoughts and beliefs when it comes to punishment and hence practice this in our real life, live in, 24/7 Master/slave relationship. Punishment should only be given if a sub deliberately starts or causes trouble or breaks rules that were put in place for her safety. Punishment should not be doled out all the time because it can have lasting effects on the sub's mental and emotional wellbeing. If you punish a sub for every slight infraction, it can start to make that sub feel worthless, instead of having the opposite effect of making them perform better.

For the 'to punish or not to punish' question, that is entirely up to the Dominant. If you know your sub has difficulties when performing certain tasks for you, but she does perform them to the best of her ability, I would say that you should be understanding and encourage her to keep trying her best. If you punish her for not being able to perform perfectly on the first or even third try, but you see that she has improved, even slightly, then punishing her for not being perfect will just add to the aggravation and disappointment she already feels inside herself.

As a true submissive, she will most likely be feeling like she has let her Dominant down by not performing the task perfectly as he asked. I will use myself as an example of this. I have epilepsy and it does have a long lasting effect on my memory. There are days when I am very slow or something as routine as the steps for making coffee are difficult for me to remember. My Padrone knows me so well and is so in tune with me that he recognizes when I am in one of these 'zones'. I have given him a cup of hot water before because I forgot to add the actual coffee to the machine! He did not punish me or yell, he actually made me feel better because I felt really stupid and was very hard on myself. He helped me laugh about it, went with me back to the machine and told me step by step what to do so that it was still my task to do, but he guided me in my time of need. There are many other examples and stories I could share, but you can see what I mean when I say punishment should fit the circumstances.

Now, if you give your sub a task like having dinner on the table when you get home from work and you find a sandwich when you were expecting a four course meal, you have to stop and think about the actual wording of the order. Did you just tell her to 'have dinner ready and on the table' by the time you get home? Or, did you say 'I want steak and mashed potatoes on the table' by the time I get home? When you give an order or task, make sure you do so in precise wording and are not vague, so there can be no misunderstandings. The more vague you are with a task or command, the more room for interpretation there is for the sub.

If your sub tends to be lazy and take the easiest way out when left with a vague order, I suggest you give her very precise orders where there is little or no room for interpretation. If she tends to be an overachiever or always exceeds your vague orders, then you are safe to continue, as you know she will always meet and beat your commands.

There are subs that love punishment or love to get punished, so they will constantly do things to make their Dominant angry and receive punishment. If you have one of these subs, I suggest you re-evaluate your relationship and how your punishment system works.

There are many different forms of punishment for both real life and cyber submissives. The main thing to remember is the point of punishment. When given, it should be done in a way to ensure the sub knows inside herself why she is being punished. It should also be done in some form or way that the submissive does not like.

As forms of punishments, a Dominant may ground, isolate, assign essays or line writing, time outs, have the slave kneel on ice/rice/pebbles, control what the sub eats, where they sleep, where they sit, or institute speech restrictions. There are many more forms of punishment, but these are the most widely used. If you notice, I left off spanking and flogging, as many subs are masochists and see these as not a form of punishment but a form of reward. So they will continue to act out just to get spanked more.

Specific Unpleasant Chore

This can include things such as cleaning the stove, cleaning blinds and windows, scrubbing the floor with a toothbrush, detailing a car, etc. The Dominant can make a list of chores and rotate through them to avoid re-cleaning a recently cleaned item. Chores assigned as punishments should not include chores that are part of the submissives normal duties. It is important to distinguish normal chores from '"punishment chores" or the submissive may start to view all chores as punishment

Sleeping On The Floor (or somewhere other then normal sleep arrangements)

This punishment is can be effective for dealing with a submissive that has become too vanilla in manner. Because of social conditioning this punishment tends to stress the position of the submissive relative to the Dominant.

Standing In A Corner

This is an old standard. It gives the submissive time to think about the infraction. The length of time can vary from few minutes to an hour or more. It is suggested that the Dominant try this punishment for themselves, to get a sense of how difficult this punishment may or may not be for the length of time in question.

Writing Assignments Of Some Specific Length

This punishment is helpful when the Dominant wants the submissive to think about or research a subject. It is recommended that this punishment be used intermittently rather then regularly to keep the act of writing from taking on a negative connotation.

Kneeling On A Hard Surface

This is a very classic punishment that combines giving the submissive time to think about the infraction with mild physical discomfort. If the length of time to kneel will exceed 20 minutes it is recommended that a full 5 minute break be given after every 20 minutes. Kneeling for too long on a hard surface can cause nerve damage. It is also good to keep in mind that some submissives may not be able to kneel 20 minutes because of physical considerations. It may be that some submissives need to do cycles of 10 minutes of kneeling and 5 minutes of rest.

Kneeling On Uncooked Rice

Kneeling on a hard surface can be made more severe by dropping a handful of uncooked rice on the floor where the submissive is going to kneel. Once the time period is done, the submissive can be instructed to clean up the rice as part of bringing the punishment to a close. This is another punishment where is suggested the Dominant try it for themselves to get a feel of the punishment. The same cautions and time limits apply to this as when kneeling without the rice. The Dominant should also be aware that the rice sometimes causes marking of the skin. Lastly, do not use instant rice as it crumbles and defeats the purpose of using rice.

Food Restrictions
Obviously some common sense is required with using food restrictions a punishment. Being sent to bed without dinner is a certainly not going to cause a healthy individual any harm. However, denying a diabetic food after they took their insulin could result in death. One suggested way to use food restrictions is to deny the submissive sweets for a period of time (days/weeks) as a punishment.

Restriction of Computer, TV Privileges, Etc.
Restriction of recreational access to things such as the computer or TV can be useful motivators when they can be enforced. The restriction can be total, where the submissive is not allowed any access to the items, or it can be limited to a certain amount of time. There is a wide range of options under this heading.

Cold Shower
A brief cold shower can be used as a rather impressive punishment. There are several points to keep in mind when using this as a punishment. First, tap water varies in temperature depending on the time of year. A small difference in temperature makes a huge difference in the severity of the punishment. Next, it is important to define what is meant by "short". Less than 5 minutes is generally quite safe for any fit person; however, 30 seconds can be quite attention getting. This is another 'try it before you use' it type of punishment.

Send the Submissive To a Room By Themselves
This one generally speaks for itself. It gives time for calming down and for reflecting. This is often a good choice when the Dom wants to avoid adding stress to a situation.

Grounding
Being restricted to home can be a relatively effective and low stress punishment. External factors greatly affect the harshness of being restricted to home. This means that the same punishment is more or less severe depending on what else is going on in the submissive's life at the time. Being

restricted when one has already bought tickets to a concert is more significant than being restricted when one has no plans.

Speech Restrictions
Speech restrictions can range from requiring the submissive to speak in third person to requiring the submissive to not speak at all for a period of time. When silence is used as a punishment it is helpful to have the submissive carry around a notebook and pen so they can convey necessary information. Requiring a submissive to speak in third person is an effective way to make the submissive aware of self-centered behavior. Many times a submissive may not be aware of how just often they refer to their own opinions and desires in casual speech.

Public Apology
Apologizing in a public forum stresses humility. The Dominant must carefully consider the reaction of those who are going to hear the apology.

Financial Penalties - Allowance Restrictions
If the Dominant controls the finances in the relationship restricting spending money can be used as a punishment. This is same as a parent withholding allowance and generally works best over shorter terms such as a week to a month. When it becomes longer than a month the punishment starts to become the norm.

Lecture
A good old-fashioned lecture can be an effective punishment. The lecture should include what specifically was wrong with the submissive's behavior and why it was wrong. The lecture should also include what the submissive should have done under the circumstance and why. If the submissive is required to maintain a physically stressful position during the lecture (such as kneeling) then the Dominant must also keep in mind cautions associated with the physical position such as time limits.

Dominant Expressing Anger
As odd as it may sound to some, the simple expression that the Dominant is angry at the submissive often carries a fair amount of punishment value. However, a fair number of submissives are inclined to view criticism and/or the expression of anger as an indication that the Dominant does not care about them. This can be nightmare of a problem and it is one that Dominants should always keep in mind.

So, in closing, always keep safety in mind, as well as the purpose of the punishment. Make sure the punishment fits the crime, it is a punishment that the sub does not like, and the lesson will be learned without lasting mental, emotional, or physical harm.

- Punishment and or discipline take precedence over any other command.
- A sub/slave must show gratitude for punishment and or discipline.
- A sub/slave must take correction gracefully and maintain a grateful presence around the house after the fact.
- A sub/slave must confess to disobedience and take responsibility even when the Dominant is not present and beg for punishment and or discipline.
- A sub/slave must always maintain the punishment position in these cases.

Chapter Twelve

Cyber/Online BDSM

Real Life play is wonderful. It's exhilarating, fun, and can be intensely erotic. Some people are lucky enough to be able to play whenever they want. Usually though, there are limitations - time, distance, obligations - which means we can't just whip up a scene whenever we feel like it. However, RL isn't the only way to explore and experience BDSM. It is often said that our most developed sexual organ is our brain and that's were cyber-BDSM comes in.

Whether or not one sees a cyber-interaction as real seems to depend upon the person's view of cyber. If a person views cyber as just another reality, then their interactions will indeed be very real to them. If a person views cyber as nothing but a fantasy play land, then their interactions will not be real to them at all.

A cyber relationship can be very real. The mind is the most influential part of a person. Cyber interactions deal directly with the mind. There are no visual inputs that can distract from the information being received by the mind. They require a greater ability to put feelings and thoughts into words. Because of this, one can create a mental and emotional bond much faster online.

Cyber offers a sense of anonymity that allows people to open up faster and deeper than they would in a face to face conversation. This enhances the feeling of emotional closeness to the person you are interacting with and strengthens the mental bond. This bond is very real to the one who feels it. The emotional responses of arguments, disagreements and such are the same for online relationships as those in reality. In some cases, the response can be more intense due to the fact that cyber interactions deal directly with the mind and heart.

The biggest danger with cyber relationships is the differing viewpoints on the reality of the relationship. If a person who views cyber as "real" becomes involved with someone who views it as "fantasy", it is a formula for disaster that ends in serious hurt. Before you get in too deeply with someone online, be it Dom or sub, make sure you both have a clear understanding of where you see the relationship leading.

It is much harder to establish and maintain a quality D/s relationship on line, especially a long term one. The average online collar lasts about 1 to 3 months.

A number of on-line Doms have a very Masterly presence, displayed only in the words they type. As the Top, the key is to make it very clear that You are in control at all times. However, that doesn't mean You are constantly barking out orders. It's more a matter of being authoritative, rather than being bossy or demanding.

Rituals are very important for all subs/slaves, but most especially cyber ones. They serve the purpose of constantly reminding the sub/slave that they exist to serve You. These can be simple or complex, and can include things like requiring them to keep their genitals clean-shaven; having certain specific duties to complete during the day, such as checking in or requiring them to ask Your permission before going out with her friends. You can also have them email you first thing in the morning or last thing at night to give you a summary of their day, their feelings about the day, and all things relevant to them. Reference the list above for more ideas that can be adapted for rituals in a cyber-relationship.

One big problem with enforcing rules in the on-line world is knowing for certain that the rules are actually being carried out. It's very easy for a sub to say they did something, but unless You have a hidden camera in their home, it's very hard to know for sure that they really did it. The same thing goes for punishments. It's impossible to spank a sub from 500 miles away. But, if the trust is there and the sub/slave really is devoted to You and the D/s relationship, they will feel a deep sense of guilt and loss if they didn't comply with Your commands. Some types of punishments for a Cyber sub/slave could be to require them to stand in the corner for a certain amount of time, to hand right an essay or a certain number of sentences and scan/email the proof it was completed to you, or to wear a butt plug for a period of time. There are a number of punishments that you can administer online and obtain proof via video or photo. Be inventive and use Your imagination. Make sure that whatever the punishment, it is something that they do not like.

Cyber is fun, safe and sexy. And you can enjoy it from anywhere you have a way to connect to the outside world.

One of the most difficult things about cyber play is that the only toy you have is your imagination. It's also one of the most exciting. This can be that grey area where fantasy and reality meet, where you can try out new things safe in the knowledge that the worst thing that will happen is the connection dropping. It can give you the confidence to explore things that you would never have tried in RL first.

With a mobile phone, you can call from, or make your sub receive the call, anywhere. Text messages are just as convenient, but have the advantage of being wonderfully discreet. Want to distract them at work? A simple SMS-ed 'Slut' should do the trick. Email isn't as interactive and immediate as other online forms of communication, but it can be particularly useful for sets of instructions, or vivid descriptions of fantasies. Write the mail, then send the text message 'Check your mail' when you know they are in no position to do so.

There are many toys a sub can easily use on himself during a cyber scene - it seems a shame not to use them. It's important to give clear instructions - and to think them through before you give them. There's no point in telling your sub to tie himself to the chair, then instructing him to go and get his nipple clamps, since things like that are impossible.

As in a RL BDSM relationship, a Top has to make sure that you have a clear list of Limits from the sub so that you don't give them instructions that will go against one of their hard limits.

Cyber to Real Life – First Meeting

In BDSM like in anything else in real life, there are people that are in the lifestyle for the wrong reasons. For those of us in the Lifestyle, trust cannot be bought with money. The only way build trust is through discussion, negotiation and time. If a partner wants money or expensive gifts up front, beware! If you want to pay for services (being dominated or Dominating), go see a professional Dominant. Do not discuss any financial matters until you have established trust and a solid relationship. If you find a good partner, and you build trust between you, make it a pleasant surprise that you are wealthy. If you flash your money before you build that trust, you will find a partner, but he or she may be with you for the wrong reasons.

The biggest danger is physical harm and/or death. Not everyone is out to hurt and kill people, but some people are. Most meetings go very well, but the dangers are very real. Submissive women are often seen as easy prey because their submissive nature can be manipulated to allow for abuse by someone who knows how. Physical vulnerability can be easily utilized by an unscrupulous person and either permanently physically harm you, or outright kill you. Make sure you have gotten references about the person you are meeting and checked them BEFORE you meet.

Don't ignore basic safety measures. There are people out there who are simply predators, and the person you are meeting may be wonderful online and the phone, but admit you don't really know him, and protect yourself until you do. Never divert from your planned itinerary on a first meeting. You planned that schedule so people could find you...if you leave it, they can't. Stay where you said you would be, when you set up your security, and resist, to the point of running away, any attempt by your partner to take you away.

Inform a close friend of where you will be and with whom. Give your friend a good description of the person you are meeting in case this is needed by authorities later. Give them the make, model and license plate number of car the person you are meeting will be driving. Leave a copy of this information out in a very visible area in your home as well, just in case it is needed by authorities later.

Set up safe calls with your friend. These are set times that you are supposed to call your friend and let them know that you are all right. If you miss your set time to call, the safe person should attempt to reach you, if they cannot, then they should be instructed to call the authorities. This goes for both doms and subs.

Numerous articles have been written about this where to meet. Every single article will stress the importance of safety. The choice of the place to meet should be during daylight hours in a public venue, where both people feel safe and at ease. Choose a restaurant or a coffee shop. You will be able to have some kind of privacy sitting at a table while you still are among people. If you choose a restaurant, make it not too expensive, but again, avoid greasy spoon places or restaurant chains (too many kids and commotion for a good discussion). A quiet, not too expensive place should do.

DO NOT PLAY! On the first real life meeting, you want to take the time to get to know your potential partner. Playing will only satisfy a sexual urge and may cloud your judgment. Realistically, many people do play on the first meeting. It is similar to the "one night stand" of vanilla relationships. Some people are only looking for a one night stand and not a committed relationship. Be sure that your desires for the relationship match your prospective partners. If play is a possibility, a play list or scene negotiation form should be used.

Remember, most meetings go very well, but there have been some incidences where the meetings did not go well and someone got hurt and/or killed. You are solely responsible for your own safety in these situations. Use common sense and you will find meeting people to be a more pleasurable experience.

Be Cautious – Predators Are Everywhere

Just as the internet culture has opened up great new ways to communicate - it has also provided a whole new way for psychopaths to con and manipulate people. Predators do exist and are a very real threat. They target both men and women of all ages and use the anonymity of the Internet to their advantage since they can be whomever they want. They look for people that are emotionally vulnerable and start to connect and manipulate them by relating to personal issues derived from problems that either occurred in the past or are currently happening. Just because we are geared towards BDSM as a community, does not mean that we are safe. We rely on honesty when dealing with our partners, but if you are just getting to know someone, do you really know that person?

Did you know that statistically speaking, 87% of profiles that contain adult content are fake? Do you really know if that person is real or not? Is the person on the other end you are telling so much real information about yourself a psycho?

I get many emails and have heard many stories mostly about subs (mostly women) that are so in love with their on-line cyber Doms, that they decide to sell everything, quit their jobs and pack up and move to where the Dom lives. But, do you really know that Dom? Why are you doing all the comprise and life changes? Is the Dom willing to come and move you? Do you have a backup plan? These are the things to think about if you are seriously thinking of making this type of move.

Before I continue, I have to say that I met my Padrone online and moved to Italy to be with him. But, he came to the USA, packed me up, paid for everything and we have been living together very happily for 1 1/2 years. There are many other tales of people that have met online and are either happily living together or married now. You have to understand though, that these are rare exceptions to the rule. I got very lucky that I met the person that completes me so well online. Most people aren't as lucky and pay a high price for not being more cautious.

Here are some tips to watch out for that can be a sure sign of an online predator:

Choosing a Victim
They study people thoroughly, and choose only those who will prove susceptible to their charms. The right victims are those that usually have a need or a void to fill, those who see something exotic in the Predator. The victim is often isolated or at least somewhat unhappy (perhaps because of recent adverse circumstances). The perfect victim has some natural quality that will attract the Predator. The strong emotions this quality inspires will make their seductive maneuvers seem more natural and dynamic. The perfect victim allows for the perfect chase.

They will Create a False Sense of Security
At first, they will just engage you in polite conversation. The seduction will begin in an indirect manner, so that you gradually start to connect with the Predator on a more personal and deep level. They will gradually move from a relatively neutral relationship to lover. They will start telling you things about their past and life that are all false, but make you relate to them on a more personal level. That is what creates the false sense of security.

They will Engage Your Friends to Use Against You
Few of us are drawn to a person that others seem to avoid. People gather around those who have already attracted interest. We want what other people want. To draw you closer and make you hungry to be possessed by them, the Predator creates an aura of desirability-of being wanted and courted by many. It will become a point of vanity for them to be the preferred object of attention. They will then 'pick' you out of the crowd of admirers. This manufactures the illusion of popularity by surrounding themselves with members of the opposite sex-friends, former lovers, present suitors, but also makes you feel extremely special because out of all the people, they chose you. The Predator may also create triangles to stimulate rivalry and make you crave them even more.

69

They will Cause You to Confuse Desire and Reality: The Perfect Illusion

To compensate for the difficulties in their lives, people spend a lot of their time daydreaming, imagining a future full of adventure, success, and romance. If the Predator can create the illusion that you can live out your dreams with them, they will have you at their mercy. They will start slowly, gaining trust, and gradually constructing the fantasy that matches your deepest desires. They will aim at secret wishes that have been repressed, stirring up uncontrollable emotions, clouding your powers of reason. The perfect illusion is one that does not depart too much from reality, but has a touch of the unreal to it, like a waking dream. They will then easily lead you to a point of confusion in which you can no longer tell the difference between illusion and reality.

This is the point that they close the net and separate you from your real life friends and family. This is the time when you will likely make a major life altering decision to move to a different state or even country, just to be with them, to live the fantasy life they have created around you. This is where you really need to step back before you make any moves and evaluate the situation in its entirety.

Are you being honest with yourself about your real desires or are they just fantasies you really do not wish to live in reality? Are you willing to sacrifice everyone and everything to make a move to be with that person? Is the Predator asking you to sever ties with everyone and only focus on them?

I have talked to many that were pulled into online illusions by what I term as Master Players. They were manipulated to the point that they either did sell everything and pack up and get ready to move, only to have something happen in the 11th hour that caused all plans to come to a stop, or they were seriously ready to start the process of trying to make that major move and something came up to bring the victim back to reality.

You have to be cautious. You have to be aware. Yes, there are many times when you take all precautions and do everything you can and still, you get burned. But the one thing that I found that was a common thread to those that did get burned was that the giving was all on one side. The victims gave and gave and the Predators took and took. There was no 50/50 sacrifices. The victim (in every case I am thinking of was a sub) was always the one that either gave up everything or was about to give up everything just to be with the Dominant.

If the Dominant wants you badly enough, they will make as many sacrifices as you to get you there to be with them. If this is not the case, then it is probably not a real situation or will not turn out to be a good situation for you.

Remember, you are priceless, so be cautious and do not make hasty decisions.

Chapter Thirteen

Collars

First, I have to say that the collar is not a fashion statement. If you really believe and want to live, what I consider, a true BDSM Lifestyle, you have to understand the meaning of a collar. Many people on the internet will give a virtual collar to anyone and then a week later, you will see they are not together anymore. In my opinion, this is not a true collaring, it's more along the lines of 'it sounds cool so let's do it'.

What is a Collar?
A collar is a device of any material placed around the neck of the submissive to signify many things. The main significance is that the sub wearing it is either taken or owned by a particular Dominant.

A Little History
Collars in historical times were put on slaves as to identify who owned them. To collar someone at the neck meant that you hold that person in ultimate control. Today's purpose in the BDSM lifestyle community collars carry many different meanings depending on the individual, but generally speaking the significance of the collar is the same - a person has control over another. One very important distinction from our historical counterpart rests in the consensual nature of the collar.

Collars were used as part of metal restraints in ancient times. However, iron collars were also used by the Romans to identify slaves and even give instructions for their return. It is likely that these historical precedents led to the association of slavery with collars in subcultures like Old Guard leather and in BDSM fiction, such as the Story of O and the Gor series.

Gay leathermen traditionally used a padlocked chain to collar their slaves. A tradition developed in some leather bars in the 1980s of wearing a collar with an open padlock to indicate that one was seeking a partner, and a closed padlock to indicate that one was in a relationship. This symbolism became less common in the 1990s as even in gay leather bars, many men began wearing collars for reasons of fashion rather than to indicate a relationship (or desire for a relationship). Also, many older leathermen were quite offended when younger men began flagging with unlocked collars.

Traditionally, the top owned the collar and locked it on his slave. Slaves or potential slaves did not collar themselves.

Types of Collars and When You Get One

Typically, a Dominant will pick the collar out for her submissive. She may involve him in the process, but normally the decision is all hers. A physical collar may be a simple chain with a padlock, a dog collar bought at the local pet store, or even a piece of costume jewelry bought at the mall.

Depending on the relationship, and their needs, a collar may lock, but it is almost equally likely that it will not. The first collar is called a *collar of consideration* and indicates that a submissive is being considered for training by a new dominant.

The second type of collar is the *training collar*. This means that a submissive and dominant have moved on to a training contract and are probably moving onward to being a long term couple.

The final collar is the one placed around the submissive's neck when the dominant *claims that submissive permanently* If it is a long term relationship, this collar would normally be lockable and made from some really durable material or metal that looks like jewelry.

There are also collars known as play collars. This collar is placed around the neck of the submissive when the dominant wants to play and protect the submissive during a scene.

In its material form, it may take many shapes. It may be a simple leather dog collar, chain, steel, a necklace, a ring, a bracelet, an anklet, or some other body decoration. It can take the physical form of a brand, a tattoo, or body piercings. Most collars seem to be designed to feel strong and secure in the relationship negotiated or formed.

Collaring Ceremonies

The ceremony may be intimate, just between the Master and slave involved, or it may be a large event with friends and family invited. If they are in an online only relationship, it may be a simple phone call, or online chat where descriptive chat is typed out. In any event, no matter where the event is held, or who attends, it should be seen as a somber event with bit of significance in our lifestyle, as a wedding is in the vanilla world.

So remember, a collar is not a fashion statement. It is a symbol of a type of deep commitment you have with your Dominant. It reminds you of the set of rules, guidelines and values you must live by while you have it on. It is a precious thing and should not be entered into lightly.

Chapter Fourteen

Polyamory in a BDSM Relationship

There are many types of BDSM relationships, from one-on-one monogamous, submissive swapping, to monogamous Poly families.

Polyamory is defined as the practice, desire, or acceptance of having more than one intimate relationship at a time with the knowledge and consent of everyone involved. The term "polyamorous" can refer to the nature of a relationship at some point in time or to a philosophy or relationship orientation (much like gender or sexual orientation). It is sometimes used as an umbrella term that covers various forms of multiple relationships; polyamorous arrangements are varied, reflecting the choices and philosophies of the individuals involved. Polyamory is a less specific term than polygamy, the practice or condition of having more than one spouse.

Polyamorous relationships take many forms and can include many different levels of intimacy. In some relationships, a couple will have a single dedicated partner with whom they share a series of affairs. Another person may be actively "single" while participating occasionally or often in the committed relationships of others. A couple may be committed to each other and to a third… or to another couple. One person who is part of a couple may be dedicated to another person who is also in a committed relationship, without the involvement their significant others. The possibilities are limited only by the needs and desires of the parties involved.

Polyamory is not something you involve yourself in because it will please your dominant. You have to desire to be in a relationship with more than one person and more than one gender. It has to come from inside you and you have to ensure that when you involve yourself with a dominant that has candidly stated that he wants more than one submissive or slave, or get involved with a couple, that you are very sure of yourself and not at all prone to jealousy.

The roles have to be clearly defined and there must be complete honesty in everything that happens. Everyone must be able to share their feelings and thoughts as they happen and prevent any bad feelings from simmering and damaging the dynamic. A submissive in a relationship with a dominant and multiple other submissives should know that all of the submissives are important and that in the end it is a privilege to serve a dominant who provides for everyone. The moment jealousy and entitlement interferes, the groups tend to break up, even when all involved cared about each other. Submission in a polyamorous situation takes even more strength than submission to one does.

If you are thinking about involving playmates or bringing on a permanent new equal as a 3rd, you have to have ground rules that all will agree to and follow. This is very important to make sure that everyone feels equal and included in all dynamics of the relationship. Open and Honest communication between all parties is a must. There can be no secrets. If you are feeling any type of negative feelings, you should tell your Dominant first and then the partner with whom you have the negative feelings as soon as possible. If you don't, it will just fester and grow until a big blow up occurs.

Be careful in picking the potential playmate/new addition. Remember, there are people out there that are very deceptive and will pretend to be one way, until they get into the relationship, then slowly try to push you apart from your Dominant. Before inviting anyone to join you, make sure you and your Dominant have deep talks about the new person and lay all of your feelings, wants, needs, desires and expectations on the table. Make sure you are very sure and have given a lot of time into getting to know the new person before allowing them closer into your family.

Overall, a poly family can be a very loving, very fulfilling experience, as long as all parties stay honest and open with their feelings.

Chapter Fifteen

Using Technology in a BDSM Relationship

Throughout the BDSM community, we see pictures of collared and leashed subs/slaves all over. I find them very enticing myself and love seeing new pictures of devoted slaves kneeling at the feet of their Master/Mistress with their leash being held. Most subs/slaves feel best and most secure when they are in close proximity of Master/Mistress. But, practicality, physical limits, family, etc., prohibits most of the leashed positions that are pictured in the images we see splashed all over the internet. How can we achieve that mental feeling of security and love when we are out in the world, or our Dominants are out, without actually, physically, being leashed?

This is where we can use technology to our advantage. If you are a Dominant and want to keep a tight leash on your sub/slave all hours of the day, make sure they have a cell phone with WiFi or Internet access. Through this, you can use many free apps to check on their whereabouts at any time you choose. Google Maps and Facebook are two of the most popular and free software you can use. Make specific rules for your sub/slave, when to check in, where and how to check in, as well as what info you want them to send when they do their check in, such as location, time estimated to be at the place, how they feel, etc. Granted, this could make some subs feel like they are being to controlled, but there are many others that would love this type of rule or control.

If you are a sub/slave and you love the feelings you get when you are on a leash connected physically to your Dominant, this is a very good alternative. If you do not wear a collar at all times, outside the house especially, ask your Dominant to pick one for you that is acceptable to be seen in public places and could be mistaken as a piece of jewelry. The weight on your neck will make you feel connected and remind you of who owns you always, no matter where you may be. If your Dominant is not with you, perform 'Check-ins' via the Facebook or Google apps mentioned above; or simply send a text message to the Dom, following the rules H/She outlined for you.

I actually call my Padrone (Master) whenever I go anywhere. If he is not at home and I need to go out, I call him before I leave, and when I reach wherever I am going. I tell him how long I think I might be there, then call him again when I am leaving. If he is at home, I call when I reach my destination, and call again to let Him know I am leaving and where else I may be going if not going directly home. I have found this gives me a sense of peace, security, and love deep inside myself, as well as giving my Padrone an added sense of security and peace of mind in knowing his slave is well. He implemented these measures because of my epilepsy, but also because He knows me so well, that he understands that any type of rule like this, that he puts in place, makes me feel that much more safe, secure, loved, and protected, especially if he is not with me.

So, the next time you as a Dominant wonder where your slave is or you as a sub/slave, wish you had that feeling of security and love that a leash gives you, try utilizing the methods I mentioned above. You will be surprised at the peace of mind and feeling of security it will bring to both the Dominant and the sub/slave.

Chapter Sixteen

How we choose to practice BDSM

As you have read, the BDSM lifestyle can take many forms, incorporating more of one thing versus another. It can be a sometimes scene or a 24/7 scene. It can and probably will, evolve into something different than what it was when you first started living the Lifestyle.

Everything that you have read is just skimming the top of the BDSM lifestyle. This guide was designed to give you an overview and help you understand or start your own journey. Now, I will tell you more of my own experience of being a 24/7 slave and a little history of how I began in this lifestyle.

I am pretty open about who I am and what I believe. I always share my own experiences when I think they will help others. I won't go into my past much, because I see the past as the past, and it is better left right where it is. Of course, it helped shape me into the person I am today, but the person I am today is so much different than I was 2 years ago.

I was at a point in my life where I was completely unhappy, with my work, my relationships, everything. I hated it. I was not in an environment that allowed me to be myself, the true me. I think I had lost the true me, my core self, many years before, because I had to hide who I was from everyone for so long.

I decided to get back in touch with my BDSM submissive roots. I had been trained for 2 1/2 years as a Gorean kajira, starting at the age of 19. Life intervened and I lost touch with BDSM and submission for many years.

I started reading and getting back into the scene via the internet around 1998. There wasn't much of a presence on the net as there is now, but it was there. I participated in many forums and advice columns as well as mentoring new people that had no clue where to start their own journey. Just as I was finding myself again, life intervened and my BDSM activities were put on hold. Over the next several years, career, kids, cancer and epilepsy, as well as the other normal trappings of life kept me away from the scene. I was lost once again.

I decided about 5 years ago that I could not continue living in that box society had forced me into. I had to break free of that shell. I felt like a walking zombie in much of my normal day to day life. I was only going through the motions of living, but not enjoying life. There is a HUGE difference from being alive and living your life.

My heart stopped beating on two occasions and I actually was dead, but was brought back. This was due to epilepsy and other circumstances. I also dealt with cancer and won. All of these things happening to me in a relatively short period of time were a HUGE wake up call. I had to get my life back on track and find my way back to being happy. I knew that BDSM, being a submissive, serving a Master that would allow me to be myself was the only way that I could be me and be happy. But, I was in a bad marriage and had two kids. How could I possibly participate in BDSM?

I found cyber BDSM again. I started devouring everything I could read on the scene, remembering my training and the feelings it brought me, of peace and comfort and joy. I started interacting with others in the same boat as myself and together, we helped each other relearn and regain our submissive sides. They had actually never been lost, just put away and forgotten, until we had a chance to bring them out again. I started participating in real life activities, non-sexual, but just around the scene to regain my sense of the Lifestyle.

After a while, I met a wonderful, smart, funny man that happened to live half a world away. He had so much wonderful advice and was so caring. He was never overbearing and you could tell, just by speaking to him, he was a natural Dominant. I talked to him and got to know him for several months before becoming his cyber slave in April of 2011.

During my time as his cyber slave, he had many rules that I had to follow. He was very flexible though and understanding because he knew I had to maintain a balance between my real life duties as well as my cyber activities. And sometimes balancing them is very hard. So over the months, we video and phone chatted, IM'd and emailed. I had as much contact with him as I could. I could never get enough. He was the one person that I felt I could just be myself. I instinctively knew I could tell him anything and he would not judge me. I completely opened up and told him about my entire life, past, present and future, wants, needs desires, hurts, dreams... Everything.

Well, in August of 2011, he flew to the USA and I returned with him to Italy, where I have been and remain very happily, his 24/7 slave.

I have grown so much in the past 1 1/2 years. I have learned to be myself again. With all of the structure, rules, and guidance that Padrone had built into our ever evolving relationship, I have never felt more safe, loved, protected, cared for, or happy in my life. We have a completely open and honest, two way communication that is the very foundation of our BDSM life. We practice more the M/s part of BDSM than the S&M, but it does govern every part of our lives. I always wear my collar, everywhere I go, with or without Him. I always follow the rules he has given me, and I know the type of answer he would give in situations that might come up in which I need to make a decision.

The form my slavery takes is perhaps different from what many of you think about BDSM slavery. I have many rules, about what I can or can't wear, who I can talk to, when and where I am allowed to go, when to check in when I am out, how long I can be out of the house, and many more. But, he has given me rules that he knows make me feel good, happy and safe. He knows without any doubts that I will follow them always. He also knows that if I do slip up and forget something, like to make coffee for him before he wakes up, there is always a reason.

He doesn't punish me for mistakes I make, because they are usually not intentional and are related to side effects from the epilepsy. When would he punish me? I would say he would punish me harshly if I ever do something deliberately, like speak to people on purpose that I'm not supposed to, or start drama, or break some other rule on purpose he has put in place.

Many of you will be thinking at this point that without punishment or correction that I can't learn from my mistakes. But I do. See, he does correct me. But it's in the form of actual correction and guidance. When I make a mistake, he will show me how to do it correctly. If I make mistakes because my epilepsy is acting up, then he will stand right beside me and tell me step by step how to do whatever the task is that I need to do. This type of correction, for me, reassures me that I am not stupid, but also helps me feel even more loved and protected and accepted by Padrone.

With this kind of Dominating or Mastering, I have grown back into the person I always wanted to be. I have gotten more in touch with myself deeply and know me very well. I don't hide anything from anyone anymore because with Padrone as my Master and life partner, I feel safe to be me.

He has encouraged me to take up writing again because he knows it's a passion of mine. He also knows how much I enjoy helping others in any way I can, so that's why I started my blogs.

I hope this answers many of your questions and helps you understand a little more about me and my background, as well as the way Padrone and I choose to practice a BDSM lifestyle.

Remember, there really is no right or wrong, and no handbook to BDSM. It's all a matter of consensual, knowledgeable decisions and the way you and your partner interpret BDSM.

Chapter Seventeen

A Brief Reality Checklist for BDSM and Submission

1. You do have rights. You have the right to walk away at any time for any reason.

2. No one can keep up a 24/7 high protocol lifestyle for long without a break for of kids, family, work and other life events.

3. No man has an erection continuously. Unless they're priapic, in which case, a doctor's visit is in order.

4. There is such a thing as PMS, and no amount of Dominance will make it go away.

5. Your cyber safeword is the off button on the front of your computer. Use it.

6. There are going to be times when you don't feel like having sex. It does and will happen. Prepare yourself mentally for it because it is just a part of life and does not mean you are a bad submissive.

7. Living a 24/7 Lifestyle is not a myth. Living 24/7 in chains, naked and kneeling is.

8. There will come a time when you see your Dominant scratching himself, belching and in need of a shower. They are only human.

9. No one understands your collar and its true meaning but you. Being proud to wear it everywhere is different than showing it off at the local market.

10. Eventually, you're going to have to take off the slave cuffs to go to some real life appointment. Get used to it.

11. People get sick. People die. Use a condom, please, unless you've been tested twice in the last year, and so has your partner.

12. Don't walk away from your friends. You might well need them later, if your dream Dominant turns into a frog.

13. If you want something, ask. Ask respectfully, ask in role, and ask in good faith. But ask. If you don't, chances are, you not going get it.

14. Just because you call yourself a slave, doesn't mean that others will agree with your definition. Be prepared to defend your views, but don't growl at others for their opinions. They have a right to them, same as you do.

15. Just because the screen name says Master doesn't mean he is one.

16. There are things you won't do in Real Life that you role played with online.

17. BDSM is not always about sex.

18. People are not always nice. You will not play at every party you attend. If you are not careful and always aware of your surrounds, you may get hurt in a non-consensual way.

19. Your Dominant is not a mind reader. You need to always be open and honest with your feelings.

20. Your Mistress is not always dressed in thigh highs and hose. A Dominant does not always have his flogger nearby. Sometimes, it's time for sweat pants and hot cocoa.

21. An argument is not the end of the world. Not resolving it, however, might be.

Chapter Eighteen

Fan Questions and My Answers

These are questions I have gotten that I thought might help you on your journey. They don't really fit a certain topic, but span across many. Thus, the reason they are put here, in their own separate chapter.

F = Fan Question or Comment
M = Me - Michelle

Question 1

F: I don't really know much about the lifestyle other than what I have read on the internet. I am 40 yrs old and for as long as I can remember I am a very passive and submissive person and enjoy being that way. I continually seek out dominant people which have at times been to my detriment. I am married to a naturally dominant man who also isn't into the scene, it's just how we are. I guess what I am asking is #1 am I too old to be suddenly getting into this? # 2 is it possible for a married couple (of 20 yrs) to suddenly adopt a D/s relationship and if so, how would we go about it?

M: Hello Natalie and thanks for coming to me for information. I love helping and guiding new people in this lifestyle.
First, I believe that age is nothing but a way to count time. It has nothing to do with our ability to change, adapt, grow or learn. I myself am 39 yrs old, so I'm very close to your age.

Has your husband shown any desire to change or enhance your relationship through BDSM? Have you talked to him about your curiosity to explore the vast variations of BDSM? That is key. There is a huge difference between a True Dominant and a dominant person. No matter your age or how long you have been married, if there is the willingness to explore and learn about BDSM, i believe it could enhance your marriage and bring you closer

I will explain. With a regular marriage, even if one partner is more dominant than the other one, for the most part you are both equals. You probably go and come as you please, wear what you want, eat what you want, go out with friends if you want and basically just tell the other one, 'Hey huni, I'm gonna go... do... whatever.....' This is how most marriages are. Well in a BDSM one, there are so many variations. BDSM does not just consist of sexual domination, bondage, spankings, or things along those lines. A huge part is one partner (in this case you) being submissive and trusting their Dominant (in this case your husband) so completely and deeply, that you have an innate desire to yield and submit to his authority, in all kinds of situations, not just sexual. Now, there are many couples that only practice BDSM inside the bedroom, but there are also those that practice more of a 24/7 type. I am one of the latter.

My Master has given me guidelines of how to dress in every occasion, how far from the house I can go without him being with me, what times I can be outside and when I have to be home. I also have many other rules, but those are just examples to help you understand.

The way to start is to first research more on what being in a BDSM relationship is. After you get a basic understanding, ask yourself, in your heart, what parts do you want to incorporate in your relationship? Talk to your husband first and make sure he would be on board? If it's more about the sexual part, you can use stockings, ties, bandanas, or other things of that nature to tie hands and feet during sex. You can also use something as a blindfold to start out with. Take it slow and get a feel of what you both would be comfortable with and want to try.

A great way is to make a list of things you want to do, may want to try, and absolutely will not do. This is called a Hard limits list. This is what you put in place before ever experimenting. Since you have been married so long, I think you know each other very well. Now, if you are looking to add the D/s (dominance and submission) part also, this is where you take orders from your Husband. He will give you things to do, rules to follow, etc. If you don't have kids at home, one of the most common rules of this type is for a slave to be naked at all times when at home and to wear a collar of some sort while in the house. I actually wear one all the time, but it's one that can be worn anywhere and nobody really knows what it is.

Question 2

F: Michelle thank you so much for taking the time to respond with such thought, you're very kind. This all sounds fantastic to me. We have touched on the subject and I suppose it is a matter of deciding how far we would like to go and as you say a bit of planning. One thing I would like to know is in a 24/7 arrangement how do you manage feelings of anger how would I express it I'm not a very angry person per se but just if it were to arise. And also if I submit completely is it discussed what I want in return all i want is attention and a feeling of being important? I imagine it to be, after all, a transaction. Again thank you so much it certainly sounds like you've had interesting life Michelle x

M: I am always happy to answer questions anytime I can.
The first one about anger is pretty much like in a vanilla relationship. Even as a slave, i do get angry sometimes, not often at all, but sometimes. It always stems from a difference of opinion or a misunderstanding between partners. But, instead of getting angry and yelling or doing the 'normal' stuff a couple would do, my Padrone and I (Padrone is italian for Master) sit down and work out whatever the problem is right there. The reason it is important to work it out as soon as something bothers you is because the longer you stew over the issue, the bigger it can come or seem. You also have to remember you are a person with your own thoughts and feelings and opinions on life. It's ok to have opposing views that aren't always the exact same as your husband's. But, you both must remember to use logic and calmly express what is bothering you. Try to do it in person and always remember to not yell, let anger take over your brain, and never disrespect the other person.

I don't know how much you have read about a D/s or BDSM relationship, but the very foundation for it is complete honesty about everything, always; complete unconditional Trust; and open two way communication. Because, without those 3 basics, how can you really submit to someone if those aren't in place? You also asked ' if I submit completely is it discussed what I want in return all I want is attention and a feeling of being important?'. I have to address this in a couple of answers. You say IF YOU SUBMIT COMPLETELY... well, in my opinion, you don't really submit to your partner unless you do submit completely. You can't submit to some stuff one minute, then turn around and act like a Dominatrix the next. That is definitely not submissive behavior. If what you meant was to become a 24/7 submissive versus a bedroom only or scene play sub, then i say the same thing. In those instances, when you are submitting yourself to your husband aka Dom, you have to give yourself entirely over to him or you won't understand the true nature and feeling a submissive feels when they totally let go. It's not easy and it does take time.

Now for the second part, once you and your husband have set rules to determine times you submit, limits of things you want to try and not try, rules and protocols, that is when you will achieve that feeling you are talking about. Because, if you think about it, in your relationship now, you don't tell him that you want to be happy or want to laugh, you just feel something at certain times and situations and that's how you feel. He can't make you feel anything. You have to attain that feeling through service to him as well as through his actions and words. For example, when I write a short article and my Padrone praises me, I get such a wonderful feeling because I know without any doubts he always means what he says. If I cook something and he doesn't like it, he tells me also. But, he does so in a nice way, not in a mean way. It does make me feel disappointment but not in him, in myself. When I know that I have done something to please him, make him feel good, or make his life easier in even the smallest way, I am happy.

I hope these answers help you forward in your journey. Please feel free to stop by anytime.

Question 3

F: Hello, I'm still kinda new to the bdsm world, and quite frankly I'm still unclear on all the responsibilities of a Dom. So if I could have a moment of your time to help me get a more educated perspective on the duties of a Dom I would greatly appreciate it. Thank you.

M: The actual responsibility of a Dominant varies on situations. It's based on what type of relationship you have with your submissive and your own beliefs and how much control you wish to exert over her. How much do you want to control your submissive and how much control does your submissive want to give you? Do you want to pick the clothes your submissive wears and regulate her entire appearance, what she eats, where she goes, her responses to other people? Or are you thinking along the lines more of being the Dominant one in the bedroom only? There are vast variables in between. The first scenario is usually reserved for a 24/7 Master/slave relationship. I am a full time BDSM slave. I am not allowed to work outside the house. My Master is the sole provider for us. I have rules about what I wear in every situation, what color range my hair can be, what type of people i can and can't talk to, rules of conduct inside and outside the house, as well as many others. I also have rules for things like what times I can go outside by myself and how far i can go away from my house by myself. But these things i gave over freely to my Master. I submitted my entire self to him and he wanted the responsibility of taking care of me. For me, the tighter and more control he has and exerts over me, is freeing. It allows me the emotional and mental freedom that my nature seeks and needs to be 100% happy. One of the main principles of a true and good Dom is that they never demand respect or submissive behavior from their partner. The partner freely gives it, always. I suggest you research keywords on the internet for things such as Dominant BDSM 101, BDSM Dominant behaviors, BDSM Dominant creeds. These will most likely be wide and varied because of the different ways and variations people practice BDSM.

Question 4

F: I have been married almost ten years and hated sex until I knew about being dominated.. I love it.

M: That's awesome! Do you get dominated only in the bedroom? How would you feel about being given tasks from your Dom to complete? Could add a different Passion and renewed spark.

F: We do it whenever wherever!!! It has been helpful! My husband does change things up often. Thanks to a few of your fans, he has just been awesome. Any other ideas we might try???

M:Have him send you tasks to do when you're out, like take off panties, write something, buy specific food for sex play layer. Or have him pick out your undies or clothes.

F: Awesome!!!! Gonna show him this message.. Thanks

Question 5

F: So I'm very much a closet submissive and I can't find a way to express it.....how do I without freaking out my partner or how do I find a dom in my area?

M: First, you should research more about BDSM, what a submissive, the different types of submissives, the different ways to practice BDSM, and grow your knowledge on the traits and responsibilities of a Dominant. Once you have studied more on the internet and books on the different thoughts of submissives, form your own thought of the type of submissive you want to be.

Make a 3 lists of limits of what you want to try, what you will not ever try, and the maybe try list. Once you know yourself and have a very good and round understanding of BDSM, approach your partner. The first thing about your partner is that they have to be naturally dominant in order to be your dominant. You don't just learn how to become a dominant if you are not truly dominant inside yourself. I would start with the sex parts and say, hey what do you think about tying me up while having sex? Or, what do you think about spanking me, adding a blindfold, adding a gag, adding a 3rd person... Whatever your list of 'want to do's' is. After you get a feel of that, then go into it deeper. If they are interested or intrigued by the thought of dominating you, then help education them further about bdsm and being a dominant.

If they have absolutely no interest of being a dominant, then if you should look for local munches in your area. A munch is a casual affair where like-minded people get together in a public place to discuss different aspects of BDSM. You can connect with more people that are into the lifestyle and then start networking from there.

Question 6

F: Hi, wondering if u can help.
New to all of this, wondering how I go about finding a dom locally.
I dont know any sites to use. I am married but curious about being a sub
Thanks for help, I am quite shy about this

M: Have you talked to your spouse about learning more about BDSM?

F: He is not interested at all

M: Then if you want to pursue it, make a fake profile that your friends and family don't know about. Then expand your knowledge by reading more about BDSM.

F: Many thanks , I made a new fb account :) appreciate it

M: Just remember to be careful who you friend. And not to give out any real information about your rl, where you live, or your contact info until you really know a person and trust them. Lots of stalkers and creepies here.

F: Can I ask , is there really such as an online DOM /sub relationship

M: yes there is. I wrote about them the other day in my blog
http://bdsmunveiled.blogspot.it/2012/11/cyber-bdsm-relationships.html

F: Oh I will do :) as completely new to this

Question 7

F: Hi I have a problem my gf wants me to fuck her and make her unconscious while doing her? What should I do and how do I do it?

M: That is called breath play if you are referring to what I think you are and I would not recommend you participate or experiment as you can do serious harm or cause death with it.

Question 8

F: I am a first time user of ben wa balls are they more pleasure or keagle work out? Are they more for pleasure and if so how far do u push them in?

M: 1. Use the restroom before placing the balls in the vagina.
2. Insert one ball at a time. Putting lubrication on the balls will help them glide in. Women have said that inserting the balls is similar to inserting a tampon. If you're not used to inserting tampons or if you're having trouble, you should lift one leg up. If that doesn't work, try inserting them while lying down.
3. Squeeze your leg muscles together and then your PC muscles together to hold the balls in. The balls should push down a little bit inside your vagina, and they will make your vagina feel "full". Much like tampons, you should eventually get used to the feeling.
4. Hold the balls inside for at least 15 minutes a day to strengthen your PC muscles. You can hold

them in for hours for a better workout.

5. If any balls slip out, wash them well with soap and water and slip them back in.

6. There are several ways to remove the balls including: jump up and down, sneeze, cough, sit and bear down as if you're having a bowel movement, insert lubricant to help them slide out, etc. If you think you might have a hard time removing the balls, then you may want to purchase balls that are strung onto a retrieval cord. In any case, it is not possible for the balls to disappear inside the body from the vagina.

To try for Pleasure:
• Rocking: With the balls inside the vagina, get into a sitting position. Rock back and forth with your legs pressed together.
• Vaginal Penetration: During sex, leave one or both balls in the vagina. The penis will move the ball(s) around, so this technique will also stimulate his penis.
• Vibrator: Leave one or both of the balls in the vagina while inserting the vibrator or using it on the clitoris.
• Retrieval Cord Balls: Use the retrieval cord to pull the balls out. Push the balls back in. This will give your vagina a good workout.

Question 9

F: Hi I'm hoping you can help me. I am familiar with the BDSM community in Seattle Washington a little and have done to a few dungeons and played very little. I'm on Fetlife, but have had little to no luck on there and don't get on much anymore. However I feel like I really want to find a Dom but I am very dominant in my everyday life and when I am approached by a man that claims to be a Dom I naturally am like prove it and I always run them off cause they are not more Dominant than me. I have yet to find a connection with someone that makes me want to submit. I am NOT into being humiliated, blood or intense pain I'm just not turned on by that. And do not want to feel inferior. I guess I'm not even sure what I'm asking but I know that I am missing something in my life and I really think that this is it and don't know where to go from here...... I need a very Dominant but respectful man. I don't need to be guided or told how to live my life this is for the bedroom only. I am a single mother of three, a two time college grad, career, home, car......I need a man to have at least that otherwise I would never respect them......any help or suggestions????

M: First of all, I do not think you are submissive at all. A submissive is someone that has an internal need to give up all control to a Dominant. They don't have requirements of what possessions that Dominant has up front. It sounds to me like you want to add kink to your vanilla lifestyle but want a partner that is as successful as you are or more so in both money and career. BDSM is not about money, careers, what you drive or where you live. The real BDSM lifestyle encompasses mind sets. The mindset of a Dominant is one that needs to be in constant control of their life, but also of those close to them. You have those Dominants that only want to be in control in the bedroom, but they demand absolute submission if only in that moment.

A submissive is someone that naturally wants to give up control, be it in the bedroom or other parts of her life. She doesn't care about the Dom's monetary attributes. She only cares about the feeling she gets when she is submitting to a Dominant.

You sound like you are at a point in your life where you have achieved many great things and are beginning to get to an age where you don't want to grow old alone or without a partner that you see as an equal, if not slightly more elevated.

I would suggest you join a vanilla dating service like match.com or some other one like that and find someone that you connect with emotionally and mentally, while they meet all of your requirements of money, wealth and status. If you find that person, you can then gradually introduce kinky play in the form of tying hands and feet, light spanking, or blind folds. You might look into buying toys to add to the bedroom excitement also.

But as far as a BDSM lifestyle goes, even in the bedroom sense only, from just your initial message, I don't think that this lifestyle would be the right path for you, especially at this point in your life. I do think that finding a sex partner that you can add some play kink in the bedroom with would be a great way for you to go.

F: I didn't mean that they had to have money etc I'm just saying that it would be hard for me to take a man seriously if he was living out of his car or wasn't in control of his everyday life. To me a Dominant has control of all those things.....and in the bedroom I want to give up all control. I want to be forced, told, made to do as he wishes.....but in order for that to happen there has to be trust and a thought of superiority. And I can't be more Dominant than my Dom.... you know??? But if I can find a stronger man than me and there is trust I can see myself completely folding for only him!

M: Wanting to submit and having a real internal need to submit are very different things. I would take time out and really search inside yourself to see what you really want and need, from the emotional and sexual standpoints. Don't force yourself into one direction or another. Once you know what exactly what you want and need, then you can decide the direction you want to travel.

F: you're right..... I def. do not have a need to submit but I def. want to...

M: That's what I mean when I say there's a huge difference. If you want to, that's more along the lines of just wanting to be kinky. If you have an internal need, you need to not be in control that is submission.

F: huh.....something to think about thank you

M: You're welcome. I don't want to discourage you from BDSM. Not at all, but do want to make sure you have a clear understanding of yourself, your own needs and expectations and wants before you start down a path you might get frustrated with or start despising because you are traveling the wrong one. If you want or need further assistance, feel free to ask me.

F: Thanks Michelle I will XOXO

Question 10

F: Just read your blog on what makes a good dom and it has me wondering ..... as a submissive who has never entered into this kind of relationship before but wants to, my safety is the most important thing, and I need to be able to trust the dom with me. Trust is a big issue and I think that you have to have trust in the dom to keep me safe. so when seeking a dom do you look for a man first to build a sub dom relationship with starting with a vanilla lifestyle and building up or do you look for an experienced dom. I'd really love fans to share how they entered into the life style i.e. if it was with a growing relationship or an experienced sub/dom

M: You can do either actually. It all depends on the Man. You have to first of all trust him and he should be a dominant male. Don't forget that Dominant is different from bully. I will post this for you. Hope you like my blog and subscribe! Many new and informative posts coming in the future!

Question 11

F: I'm a single uk man who is a bdsm virgin, I'm 38 and at the point of my life where every day I get kinkier, I've read the forbidden books the shades and countless overs and I love the whole sub Dom idea of things, I don't have trouble meeting women but when it gets down to things I'm finding it hard to get aroused in a vanilla situation, I don't see myself as shy but scared to share my needs with a woman in case she thinks I'm strange! Really need help, frustrated ain't the word!

M: Hello. I don't think it's strange that you don't get aroused in a vanilla situation. Many men don't. But, what you do need to do is research and grow your actual knowledge of BDSM from not only a Dominant view, but also a submissive. Knowing both sides will help you have a better feeling for what a sub feels and goes thru, but also help understand bdsm as a whole. Make a list of the different aspects of bdsm that you would like to explore, examples are bondage, pony play, golden showers, doggy play, diapers, spanking, collar and leash, flogging, piercing, and there a whole lot more. Compile 3 lists. One that you like, one that you will never try, and one that is a maybe. with that knowledge, go to fetlife and utilize other sites, maybe even google munches in your local area to start going to, and start mingling with real life people that practice bdsm. Do not be scared to share that you are a newbie, and just be open and honest. That should help you.

F: Wow thank you Michelle for your time all taken on board

M: You are most welcome. Glad to be of help.

Question 12

F: Pls help, fairly new to the scene, married, but hubby has made it clear he doesn't want to dominate me in any way shape or form, but my need to be a submissive is getting greater the more I read up on it, although I love my husband, I feel I need a Dominant in my life as well, not necessarily for sexual play, how would I go about finding an online Dom to tick my boxes? Thanks xx

M: I have two schools of thought. If you still love your husband and don't want to possibly mess up your marriage, be truthful with him about your need to be dominanted. If he doesn't want to do it, then ask him if he would mind an online only relationship with a Dom that will hopefully feel the need. The first thing you have to realize is that you won't connect with just any Dominant. You will talk to many online and might find one that likes and wants the same things as you do and had the correct attitude that suits yours. If you don't want to involve your husband, make a fake profile with all fake information and search on FB for the keywords bdsm. There are many pages that allow hookups and you can also add other people with similar interests.

F: Thanks so much Michelle, never thought of setting up a fake profile, he's made it crystal clear he won't dominate me, pity there's not an fb page called Dom's r us!! There's so much info out there I don't know where to start looking! Xx

M: Start with the fake profile and liking all of the BDSM related links you can find. Then friend people that you think might be interested in the same things as you are or find groups about education in BDSM also.

Question 13

F: I am a complete newborn. I have teetered on the edge of delving fully into the lifestyle for awhile and feel it is time to jump, so to speak, how would you suggest I ease my way into it???? I am adventurous to say the least when it comes to the sex part. It's the trust I have issues with. I mean to fully subjugate yourself wouldn't have to trust the person not to go farther than your limits?? Like I said before I am totally fresh. I would appreciate your advice but would also like to keep quiet about who I am.

M: Be cautious, and grow your knowledge. Read what you can on the internet or find books that interest you. I suggest you stay away from erotica fantasy books as they don't depict the real life of a slave or submissive. Keep a running list of things you like and things you don't, but also of things that you are on the fence about. This can be transferred later into what is known as a Hard Limits or Limits list that you will share with your Dominant partner or partners.

Question 14

F: I just recently revealed to my husband of 11 years my craving for the BDSM life style. I have a very dominate personality in our marriage, but I want to be dominated by him in the bedroom. I wish to explain to him what I need so that he can feel comfortable in taking control and my submission without fear. I am afraid I will run him off if I can't get him to understand. I can see the Master I need in him and the love of my life he has always been. I don't want to lose either! Please help me.

M: You have to keep an open and honest conversation going with him about what your needs and feelings are. Get him to open up and help him understand exactly what you want from him. Introduce him to more of what a Dominant in BDSM does and is and the parts that you crave from him. There is such a wide variety that it will be good to narrow down exactly what you each want and expect from the relationship, but after you have done your homework and research.

F: I want to say thank you! My husband and I have talked more about what I wanted and about my limits. To my surprise he was more than willing to help fulfill my needs. We are starting slow with just commands and spankings for now until he is more comfortable with his new role. Then I hope to grow from there. Thank you all for your advice! It means the world to me!

Question 15

F: Hi..I am a newbi.. This has interested me for months. I have been talking with a switch who has decided to become a Dom. He want to do video chats n visuals ...is training online like this normal? n how do it really work if it isn't a handle on training? This is a little scary since I do not live chats ..but am willing to do it live chats..can you please guide me ???? I know I have to trust that all of this is privy only to him n me..
Thanks

M: I will tell you yes it is a normal process. I will advise before anything like this is done please get to know this man and inquire about him. There are a lot of people out there that are not who and what they say they are. I am not a fan of the virtual training and I do not just trust anyone. I would take your time and talk with others before making a decision like this. It is in your best interest to do this.

Question 16

F: I'm a sub by nature and my hubby requires submission in every aspect of our relationship except sex it's the one place he wants to be equals or all ideas to come from me but when I give ideas I think he takes them as a joke but we have discussed bdsm in sex play but we are at opposite ends of the spectrum on how we think it should work and we are having difficulty finding a middle ground to start on. Any advice would be most welcome.

M: Make three Limits lists – One hard (which means things you never ever will do or want to try); Soft (Things you are curious about but not exactly sure if you would like it or not); and one that contains all the things you really like and want to do more of. This should give you both a better understanding of what you like and path for future exploration.

Question 17

F: Hi, I live in a place where bdsm is really unheard of! But I have always had these feelings I've never understood I'm still confused! Even when I was a child playin mummy's n daddy's it was weird feeling like to be controlled was good... I can't explain it.... Is that good? So I'm looking to see what it is I feel if it's for me! Do you know anyone I can chat with to try understand me? I know I'm sub in my heart.

M: I would say read up on Daddy Doms or find sites that are in to Babygirl Daddy Dom play if that is the type of BDSM you are more comfortable with. There are so many ways and varieties of bdsm, you have to find what you like. The best way is reading and research. You can also join a community called Fetlife.com. It's for all different types of fetishes and kink lifestylers.

Author's Note

Thank you for reading BDSM Basics for Beginners. I hope this helped you further along in your journey into the beautiful and fulfilling world as a BDSM Dominant, Switch, Submissive or Slave.

If you would like to further your education and knowledge, I encourage you to visit me on the internet at:

Blog – www.bdsmunveiled.com

Google+ - plus.google.com/u/0/112450374015048658322

Facebook - www.facebook.com/MichelleFegatofi

Tumblr – michellefegatofi.tumblr.com

You can leave comments, ask me questions, or participate in forums with other people exploring BDSM as well.

100

24733715R00063

Made in the USA
San Bernardino, CA
07 February 2019